how to be a happy mum

Also by Netmums and available from Headline

Feeding Kids: The Netmums.com Cookery Book
with Judith Wills

how to be a happy mum

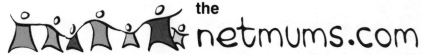

the netmums.com

guide to stress-free
family life

with Siobhan Freegard

headline

First published in 2007 by
HEADLINE PUBLISHING GROUP

6

Cataloguing in Publication Data is available from the British Library

Paperback 978 0 7553 1606 9

Typeset in Clearface Regular by Palimpsest Book Production Limited,
Grangemouth, Stirlingshire

Printed and bound in Great Britain by
Clays Ltd, St Ives plc

Headline's policy is to use papers that are natural, renewable and
recyclable products and made from wood grown in sustainable forests.
The logging and manufacturing processes are expected to conform
to the environmental regulations of the country of origin.

HEADLINE PUBLISHING GROUP
A division of Hachette Livre UK Ltd
338 Euston Road
London NW1 3BH

www.headline.co.uk
www.hodderheadline.com

Contents

Introduction

Remember when you thought you were so well prepared to be a mum? You had devoured and read every single line of your pregnancy and birth book. You'd got pretty much the entire contents of Mothercare in your house – all that wonderful, gorgeous new baby stuff . . . a crib with frilly lining, cosy soft blankets, new curtains in the newly decorated nursery, the best pram you could afford, drawers full of the cutest imaginable baby clothes and all sorts of gadgets, kit and caboodle that you hadn't quite worked out what to do with yet: slings, baby baths, rockers, baby gyms. You'd got the best for little baby in terms of the most snuggly nappies, the softest Babygro and the safest cot . . .

If there was anything you weren't sure about, you'd bought or been given The Baby Books. The ones that tell you how to feed, bathe, clothe, hold, put, push and pull your baby in pretty much every conceivable circumstance. And if you couldn't find the magic answer in the books, there's also the World Wide Web, with untold pages of advice about baby and childcare.

And then the baby came. That real live wriggling, crying, beautiful baby. There were no mysteries any more, no wondering . . . you'd crossed the line, come through the tunnel, found yourself on the other side of the fence. So that was that then. Job done. You're a mum.

This book is about what happens next . . .

With hindsight, you laugh in the face of your old self, who thought she was prepared for this. You actually feel less prepared than if you were given a brand new sports car on your thirteenth birthday, put in the middle of the M25 and asked to drive home. Or dropped by helicopter at the base of the north face of Mount Everest and asked to climb to the top. Or asked to sail single-handed around the globe, beating Ellen MacArthur's record. And the most bewildering thing is that no one else seems to think this is a lot to ask! Everyone else thinks that you are perfectly capable of doing the job, even though you've never passed your driving test or climbed a small hill or stepped foot on a boat other than a car ferry.

Your husband goes back to work and the rest of the world seems to assume it's back to business as usual. People start asking normal things, such as, 'What did you do this week?' or, 'What are you doing this weekend?' or even, 'So when are you going back to work?' Except that, for you, life feels far from normal. You didn't *do* anything this week, you just, well, got through it. You're not *doing* anything this weekend – except the same as you do all week. Normal? You feel sure life will never be normal again! You begin to realise that becoming a mum is the beginning of the longest journey you have ever undertaken, both emotionally and physically.

Ask the Netmums:

What was the biggest shock for you about becoming a mum?

The sheer frustration and effort required to get ready to leave the house. No longer could I shove on a pair of trainers and grab my keys! Outings have to be planned with military precision and getting everyone ready takes so long. Three years down the line it is still driving me bonkers!
Sarah Jo

The fact that people automatically assume you know what you are doing! The midwives at the hospital were a nightmare. Sam is my first baby and nobody tells you how to do the basics. I remember getting frustrated because I couldn't burp him (he was later diagnosed with reflux). When I asked the midwife how to do it, the helpful answer I got was, 'You just do it.' There is this little person totally reliant on you and no instruction manual!
Michelle

The lack of sleep. I know people warn you, but I really wasn't prepared for it. I was breastfeeding and up every two to three hours for almost six months. I never got a full night's sleep until my son was eighteen months old. I spent a lot of time being excessively tired, grumpy and very short-tempered. It put a real strain on my relationship with my husband. It was absolutely amazing when my son started sleeping through; it was like a weight had been lifted from the house and everything started falling into place.
Irina, Ayrshire, mum to Max, 2

What shocked me was how much I adored my daughter from the very first second. I really didn't know how I'd feel but I was utterly stunned and still can't get my head round how amazing she is and just how much I love her.
Katherine, Nottingham, mum to Daisy, 20 months

I think the biggest shock was when it suddenly dawned on me (after about four years) that it was actually a permanent situation. I kind of expected that all the turmoil, the constant worry, keeping them from danger, the loss of spontaneity and loss of self, etc. was a temporary thing and that soon I'd be going back to my old self. Then one night it hit me that this was *it*. There was no going back to the way things were before – *ever*.
Claudia, Bedford, mum to Sophia, 5 and Mia, 3

Everything. I went from working full time and going out three or four times a week with groups of people to not working at all, not being able to go out and feeling that the only person in my life other than my darling daughter was my other half. I became really clingy and horrible. The sleep issue was hard at first as well. Becoming a mum hit me like a ton of bricks. Everything had to change, seemingly overnight. No matter how much you feel you are ready for motherhood, I don't think that you have any idea what it will be like until you actually do it.
Lisa, Hull, mum to Jamie, 6

One of the biggest shocks for me is how much I've changed – somebody who was once confident now questions everything and I feel like I've lost *me* somewhere.
Susan, Dudley, mum to Emma, 10 months

For me, it is the constant worry and guilt that I experience. I feel such incredible guilt about everything I do . . . Do they eat healthily, do they have too much fruit, is that nappy digging in, does one child get more attention than the other, should they go to nursery and socialise or am I just getting rid of them, etc., etc., etc.? It never stops!

I was also not prepared for the nightmares. Loads of mornings I wake up and refuse to go into my son's bedroom until I hear him make a sound. I am paranoid he could have died in his sleep. I think about the 'what ifs' so much I think my head will explode. My favourite saying is, 'I wish I could see into a crystal ball, know they were going to be OK and then relax!' But that's not realistic. I just have to try to get on and do the best I can. I wouldn't swap it, though, not for the world!

Sarah, Scarborough, mum to Hermione, 2 and Locksley, 1

Babies don't start sleeping through the night at six weeks. Your house is never going to be really tidy again. Your body doesn't ping back into shape and it doesn't look like it's going to. You'll struggle to get an hour to yourself in the bathroom; you'll fight for a lie-in; hangovers aren't worth it any more; Saturdays are no easier than Mondays; and dads don't go off sex like mums.

And just as you think maybe you are getting to grips with things, everything changes: the first teeth start waking the baby just as he has started to sleep through; the baby starts crawling, then toddling; the end of your maternity leave looms; you go back to work; you discover you are pregnant again; the arrival of the new baby upsets your toddler. Your house is even more untidy than it was before, your jeans are even tighter, your circle of friends even smaller, your job even harder to find time and energy for.

And yet, the period of having young children is supposed to be the happiest time of our lives. Ask anyone of our grandparents' age and they'll tell you to make sure you enjoy every minute, as it all passes by so quickly. But sometimes a single day can feel like a lifetime.

This book, just like the Netmums website, came about because we know exactly what it is like to be a miserable mum. We know how it feels to want, so badly, to be a perfect mum, but to feel you are failing at every turn. We know how it feels when you look about and think that every other mum seems to know instinctively what to do, while you sometimes feel you are barely coping. The truth is that no one finds it easy being a mum. It isn't easy! Everyone has difficult times and stressful times. But there are solutions. There are ways of coping with these stresses and of *enjoying* being a mum to young children. It *is* possible to be a good mum and a happy mum. And it's important for mums to be happy. Mums are the centre of the family and the centre of the home. If mums are happy, children will be happy and dads will be happy; in turn, this will spread to entire communities. This book looks at the main barriers to our happiness. Taking each one in turn, we examine new ways of looking at the issues mums face and new ways to break down those barriers.

See how many from this list of the top ten stressors you recognise in yourself:

1. Friends (or lack of them)
2. Children's behaviour (including sibling rivalry)
3. Sleep
4. Relationships
5. Money and working
6. Childcare
7. Clutter and chaos
8. Lack of me-time

9. Depression and stress
10. The unexpected (or the stuff life throws at us)

It might be that one or two are affecting you this week, but it was something else last week and it'll be something else next week (or next year). If you have a new baby, you may be all-consumed by sleep (Chapter 3), but as that sorts itself out, you might find you are arguing with your partner more than usual (Chapter 4). Then you find you have money worries, so you need to look at whether you should go back to work (Chapter 5) and the childcare you will need (Chapter 6). This book takes each of these problems in turn and examines them and the issues surrounding them. We offer an insight into and understanding of these problems and why they are so common amongst mums. We offer practical solutions, coping strategies, new ways of looking at things and, crucially, we draw on the experience and wisdom of many other mothers who have been through these issues and lived to tell the tale.

Meet the Team

Siobhan Freegard

Often the best advice, information and support in the job of being a mum come from other mums. Only other mums who have been through similar experiences can truly understand how being a mum can take you to the outermost limits of your emotional and physical strength, or how your day can swing many times over from total frustration and despair to overwhelming love and pride.

I drew this book together based on my own experiences and those of thousands of other mums I have met through Netmums. This book is filled with insight, advice and support from mums from up and down the country: mums of babies, mums of toddlers and mums of older children; mums of boys and mums of girls; working mums and stay-at-home mums; rich mums and poor mums; everyday, wonderful mums. Mums like you.

I am also privileged to have been able to draw on the support of our wonderful team at Netmums: Sally Russell and Cathy Court, who have been by my side since Netmums was just a gleam in our eyes. Emma, Donna and Nikki, who supported me in putting this book together in so many ways and every member of our team who makes Netmums what it is. And my sincere thanks to each and every mum who is quoted in this book: your generosity and openness will reach many new mums who are following in our footsteps.

I'd also like to introduce Christine, Liz and Elisabeth. I have been fortunate to have had their professional input and advice while writing this book and their wisdom and expertise gives credence to our own on-the-ground experiences.

I left Ireland, on the first boat after my eighteenth birthday, for the bright lights and big city of London. I got an office job and studied for a business diploma at evening classes. I worked my way up the corporate ladder to become marketing director for one of the Wembley Group of Companies. I married Paul, an Englishman, and we had our first child in 1996. Having a baby turned my world upside down and my priorities on their heads. Although I did go back to work, within two years I realised that I wanted to spend more time at home and I took a year off from my career. Ten years later I am still on 'my year off'.

Netmums came about from my own experiences of being a new mum, which I later learned are pretty much the same experiences as all new mums. I now have three children: Sean aged 10, Aisling aged 7, Aran aged 4 – and Solo the baby-substitute puppy.

Christine Bidmead, MSc, RGN, RHV

Christine Bidmead is married with three grown-up children. Having previously qualified as a nurse and midwife, Christine is a Registered Health Visitor (RHV) who has worked for many years in a variety of communities, both rural and urban. Over the last four years she has been with the Centre for Parent and Child Support at the South London and Maudsley NHS Trust, where she is a training facilitator for the Family Partnership Model. She trains health visitors, school nurses, teachers and other frontline professionals, volunteers and parents.

As well as her professional qualifications, Christine undertook a three-year counselling diploma, which gave her skills that significantly changed her practice. Her last health-visiting post saw her initiating and running parenting programmes and a sleep clinic for under-fives. She developed within her community a group of parents able to run the parenting programmes alongside her as well as supporting each other. Out of this grew the local trailblazer Sure Start programme in Edmonton Green, North London. During this time, her NHS Trust awarded her three discretionary pay points for exemplary practice.

Christine has also published widely in the *Community Practitioner Journal* and has co-written the Community Practitioners' and Health Visitors' Association (CPHVA) publication *Positive Parenting: A Public Health Priority*. Her other publications for the Family Partnership Model include co-writing the handbook and training manual. Working with parenting magazines and freelance journalists, Christine has had input into publications such as *Mother and Baby*, *Pregnancy and Birth* and *Practical Parenting*. She has recently gained an MSc in Community Health and has been involved in research, liaising closely with universities in order to facilitate the acceptance of the Family Partnership Model as part of core health-visitor training.

Christine has given numerous presentations about her work and that of the Centre for Parent and Child Support both nationally and internationally. She is computer literate and moderates two e-groups: one for health visitors with a special interest in parenting and family support, and another for the Association for Infant Mental Health (AIMH). She founded the former group, which numbers some 200 practitioners, and continues as an active committee member, supporting practitioners with the most up-to-date research, policy and practice developments. She has worked closely with the National Family and Parenting Institute, the Parenting Education and Support Forum and the NSPCC. She is a committee member of AIMH and a trustee of Action for Prisoners' Families.

Elizabeth (Liz) Ann Andrews, MA, RGN, RM, RHV, Adv. Dip Counselling

A British Association of Counselling and Psychotherapy (BACP) accredited counsellor committed to providing a service to meet the individual needs of client groups, Liz's background is in nursing. She is qualified as a general nurse (RGN), midwife (RM) and health visitor (RHV). During the twelve years to January 2002, she worked in the community as a health visitor, and completed her own research (Master of Arts degree) into communication issues with an ethnic minority group. This time included four years on secondment to the University of Reading, where she took part in a research project commissioned by the Department of Health. The project sought to deliver therapeutic care to women vulnerable to post-partum difficulties via the person-centred counselling approach. Liz co-authored *The Social Baby* (July 2000) that sets out to show parents and professionals how babies communicate from the moment of birth, using behaviour as their language of communication. It is hoped that, by understanding a baby better, a deeper sense of relationship will ensue. Liz is now working as an independent counsellor in the private sector.

Dr Elisabeth Hopman

Dr Elisabeth Hopman is a part-time GP in Chiswick, London, and a mother of three children: Alexander, 11, Madelaine, 9 and Cecelia, 6. She came to study medicine as a mature student at The Royal Free Hospital in Hampstead after qualifying there first as a nurse. Prior to this she worked for the New Zealand Foreign Office in Brussels and was a keen linguist. She is married to a hospital consultant and lives in Harrow on the Hill.

As a mother of three young children Dr Hopman has a personal understanding and insight into the specific issues facing mothers and she has a particular interest in supporting mothers during this time in their lives.

1 Why Mums Need Mates (and How to Find Them)

Mum-friends are lifesavers. They are our daily companions, our confidantes. They give moral support at new toddler groups and share our children's ages, stages and phases. Our children cut teeth together, learn to walk together, fall over together, play together and finally start playgroups and even school together. We go to each other's children's birthday parties and watch each other's children grow up.

More than everything else, friends with children the same age are our sanity savers. Only other mums with children of the same age truly understand what we're going through and only they want to share intimate and graphic details of our children's lives. Each age carries its own trials and joys, from babies' feeding and sleeping issues to how to get a place in your chosen primary school. And yet, few of us have a ready-made social circle of friends with babies and small children.

These days people move about so much more. Our best friends, our school or university friends are scattered across the country, the continent and the world. We email, maybe text, send birthday cards and perhaps see each other when we go home at Christmas or on other occasions. Sadly, these friends aren't around on a wet Monday for coffee and baby talk, or an 'I'm not just a mum' glass of wine on a Friday night.

Workmates or social friends are the ones you went out with for dinner or drinking and dancing. Many haven't (yet) got children of their own; these are the friends who turn up with flowers and teddies and designer baby clothes when your baby is born. Then they want to know when you can go on your first post-pregnancy big night out. These are the friends whose calls get fewer and farther between as they realise you aren't going to turn back into your old self. That reckless, do-and-be-damned, good-time girl has become a boring mum. They never quite understand that you will turn into a pumpkin if you stay out past 10.30, never mind midnight. Others who already have children are busy juggling and adapting to their own new lives as mums. While meeting in town for cocktails was easy pre-children, the logistics of dragging buggies and babies to a chaotic meeting up in a coffee shop hasn't got the same appeal, despite your best intentions.

We probably don't have our family to fall back on either: statistically we are less likely to live near our extended family – our sisters, our cousins and our own mums. Netmums' research[1] shows that, whereas in the 1960s half of mums with young children lived near their extended families, now only a third of us have family living near by. The days of having a big local family where everyone lives round the corner from each other and helps each other out are gone. No longer do we have heaps of relatives and family friends happy to hold the baby or have the toddler round for the day.

(1) Netmums' research, *Mums Then and Now*, published 2006

Also, the majority of us have moved away from where we grew up, so our school and teenage friends aren't there to share and support us through this next life stage.

Mums are having babies later too. Rather than our peer group having babies at about the same time, our babies are stretched out over the years, and our group of friends is stretched out all around the country. Add this to the fact that, with so many mums at work, we are much less likely to meet and get to know the young families living in our street.

All of this has led to a loss of good old-fashioned community, a community in which you know your neighbours, bump into half a dozen people you know on your way to the shops and can pop in for a bit of advice from your friend in the local chemist. This is true to the extent that recent Netmums' research[2] showed six out of ten mums don't have good friends in their local areas that they can rely on. That's a lot of lonely mums out there!

Ask the Netmums:

Do you ever feel lonely?

I'm a stay-at-home mum. After my son was six months old, everyone else seemed to be back at work. For a long time I didn't know any other mums. Even now I have one good mum-friend and another couple of mum-friends, but none of them is less than four miles away, and sometimes it would be nice to know someone whose house I could just pop round to!
Anon

I'm very lonely as a mum. I'm a first-time mum, and because I work I never get to meet any other mums and kids.
Susan, Dudley, mum to Emma, 1

(2) Netmums' research, *A Mum's Life*, published 2004

All the time, when my other half was at work and my daughter was a baby, I felt terribly lonely. I was so desperate to meet someone else who understood how I felt and what was going on, especially as everyone kept telling me how well I was coping and inside I was falling apart. I think it was the loneliness that caused me to feel that way. Once I was able to go back to work and see people again, I felt a lot better and was able to cope again.

Lisa, Hull, mum to Jamie, 6

Maybe I'm weird or I just like my own company, but I've never felt lonely! It was just me and my little one for the first year of her life. I wasn't working and we lived in another country, so there were no friends or family around. It didn't really bother me. Now we're back in England and I'm a stay-at-home mum, but I still don't get lonely. We do things every day either for her (Tumble Tots, etc.) or me (gym) and I have to say I love her company. I don't really have a strong need to interact with other mummies.

Helen, Congleton, mum to Willow, 3

Being a mum without any family around or any friends is very, very hard. When my three kids were all young, aged four and a half years, two and a half years and six months old, I found everything so exhausting. It would have been so lovely to have a friend around, or someone to help ease the load a bit. There were many times when I'd burst into tears from the exhaustion or from the loneliness. Never having any adult conversation was dreadful. I used to be a confident, chatty person, but now I'm quiet and have little self-confidence. I found that the local toddler group was extremely cliquey. I'd try to strike up a conversation with someone who was usually sitting alone, but never managed to get anything other than 'yes' or 'no' from them. I often thought it would have been a good idea if the group leader got everyone to sit in a circle and get all of the mums to talk about themselves: how they are finding it being a mum, their likes and dislikes . . . anything really, just to get the mums talking to each other rather than their selective group of friends.

My kids are a lot older now. The mums at the school are still cliquey, I still have no family around to babysit or help out and I have just one friend.

Christine, Northamptonshire, mum to Holly, 12, Chloe, 9 and Jack, 8

I know all about being lonely . . . and I wish I didn't. I hate being on my own. I know I have my babies but I do miss adult company. I am married and that is a blessing, I know, but I only see him for an hour or so in the evenings, as he works so much, and it can be a long old day on your own.

Emma, Swansea, mum to Bethan, 3, Ffion, 2 and Ryan, 11 months

Being at home with small kiddies (three years old and ten months) can be a very lonely life. My husband works shifts so we don't live a normal Monday to Friday 9 to 5 kind of life. Weekends seldom break up the sameness. It's so tough. In the past I'd keep telling myself that when I could drive, things would be better. When the children are both at school, things will be better.

In today's world, many of us do not know our neighbours. We might walk to the local shops without passing anyone we know or even without speaking to the shop assistant other than to say 'please' or 'thank you'. We hear it said, and I believe it is true, that the loss of the sense of community means that fewer and fewer of us are surrounded by people we know. I've lived in my house for three years and have never set foot in either of my next-door neighbours' houses. Netmums helps us to feel there are others out there in the same boat – that we all need/crave company and want to help other people who feel lonely.

I know that when I am lonely/bored, I find lots of other things that are wrong in my life to kind of prove I am a worthless individual. That good old 'self-fulfilling prophecy'! So do I have a cure? Nope! I think for me it comes down to living for the moment – really living for now and not for 'when I have friends' or 'when I get my life back'.

I have worked out how long I have to go before we have a nappy-free house and before I get a few hours' me-time every day. When I realised that could be maybe just a year away, it changed the way I think. In a year's time, this stage will be over – I'll never have this again, where I am with my children all the time. A year flies by so quickly. I want to make sure I am conscious of every moment instead of wishing things were different. The situation hasn't changed; my attitude has.

I have found local groups to go to and if I go, I try to sit back and look at the cliques to see if I really want to be part of any of them. If I do, then I make an effort. If I think, 'Can't be bothered', then I just go for the cup of coffee.

I still get days when I clock watch – but I used to do that when I worked in an office. I still get days when it seems like everyone on earth is out doing something and we are in doing nothing! I still want to achieve all my ambitions, but I'll

have to wait contentedly for the right time to come, rather than be constantly frustrated by motherhood turning me into . . . well . . . a mother!
Fiona, Surrey, mum to Christopher, 3 and Katie, 1

Before I had our son, I had a huge circle of friends. I was your typical girly girl, out on a Friday night, rolling in at all hours, up on a Saturday out shopping until my feet ached and lounging about on a Sunday watching the *EastEnders* repeats and lying in bed until all hours of the day. During the week I went to the gym three times and to two aerobics classes with friends of mine – what a laugh we had! After work we would go for a drink and talk about all things girly and bitch about our bosses. I wore nice clothes, and made an effort to look nice and smell great.

Six months later I sit here with you girls as my only source of contact. I didn't realise that kids could make you feel like the loneliest person in the world. When you need all the support you can possibly get, people turn their backs on you, giving the excuses: 'I thought you would be busy', 'Not sure what time to call', etc., etc. Why don't they understand that inside you are tearing yourself apart wondering what you have done wrong, when the only thing that has changed is that you have become a mother and perhaps if they took the time to call they would find out what your true feelings are and what your routine is so they will know when to call or pop over for a cuppa?

I still, to this day, feel very lonely – a feeling I never thought I would experience. My circle of friends is my partner and his mum and dad. That is it. It couldn't get any worse, to be honest!
Dyanne, Fife, mum to Luke, 10 months

I know I'm lucky to be a stay-at-home mum but the loneliness has been a shock.
Sarah, Essex, mum to Samuel, 2

I hate the school run. It is just so awful. I have another fourteen years to go (my youngest is two). To be honest, the thought of standing in the playground or dropping off and being ignored brings tears to my eyes. I have spoken about it to my closest mummy friend and I know that she feels the same – surely there is more to life than this! At the moment I am feeling it very badly, as I have pick-ups at 12, 1pm and 3pm – aghh! It is the loneliest feeling in the world standing in the playground to the side of all the cliques.
Julia, West Kent, mum to Finn, 6, Rory, 4 and Aidan, 2

I moved from my home-town five years ago and still feel like an outsider. I feel really low at times and think, 'What is wrong with me?' My eldest has just started school, so I am making a real effort to speak to other mums, but only a couple speak and the rest are all in their little groups. The couple of friends I have made also moved here from other places and have said that it took years for them to make friends and mainly it happened through their kids, but at this rate I don't know if I will ever make any more friends!
Sharon, Cornwall, mum to two, 4 and 1

So, you go one of two ways. You stay at home, hoping that someone will phone or call. When they don't – when you realise that hours, days and weeks can go by without anyone getting in touch – you start to get lonely, and a bit down. You may find that that causes you to retreat further into your shell. This is a long, lonely and dark road to be on and ultimately can drive anyone around the post-natal depression bend. The other path to choose is one where you start to build a new life for yourself as a mum. It's a bit like being a new girl at school or a new girl in the office – for a while you feel like an outsider. You feel you don't quite fit in. Like anything worthwhile in life, building a new life as a mum takes time and effort, but it is so very important.

Just one mum-friend is enough to make a massive difference to your life. The two of you can form a common bond and can push your prams side by side – you against the world. You can go on adventures, trying out all the local parks, play areas and groups. You can check out how baby-friendly the local cafés and shops are. You can mind each other's babies while you make that overdue trip to the dentist or even have a quick haircut. Two mum-friends are even better than one. Together you are a little gang – a circle of friends.

The scientific argument for friends

Numerous studies have shown that friends aren't a luxury but a necessity. We *need* social relationships in order to live happy and healthy lives. Here are a few examples from a wide selection of scientific studies:

- In Sweden, more than 17,000 people between the ages of 29 and 74 were studied for six years between 1981 and 1987. The people most socially isolated were almost four times more likely to die prematurely during this period. Controlling for other factors, such as age, health-behaviour or prior health status, did not change the results.[3]
- In California, a study of 7,000 people published in 1979 showed

(3) Orth-Gomer, K. and Johnson, J.V., *Social Network Interaction and Mortality: A six-year follow-up study of a random sample of the Swedish population*, 1987 (J Chron Dis 40: 949–57)

that those who lacked social and community ties were two to three times more likely to die in the nine-year follow-up period, regardless of age, health, gender or health practices or physical health status. In fact, those with close social ties and unhealthy lifestyles lived *longer* than those with poor social ties and healthy living habits (of course, those who had close social ties and a healthy lifestyle lived the longest).[4]

◆ And if living longer isn't a concern, then this one might be for you: in a 1997 study, 276 healthy volunteers were exposed to the common cold virus. Those with the most diverse social networks were the most disease-resistant; only 35 per cent of those with six or more close relationships caught the cold compared with 62 per cent of those with three or fewer social relationships.[5] So the more friends you have, the less likely you are to get a miserable winter cold![6]

How to make friends with other mums

This section is not just for new mums. If you are a mum with older children, or a second- or third-time mum, for heaps of reasons you can still find yourself not having quite broken into the world of mums. You may find yourself at the pre-school or primary school gates, standing alone while everyone else seems to know each other.

It's a bit like re-entering the dating game. And just as with meeting men, it's highly unlikely that your new friends will come knocking on your front door asking you out to play. The difference, of course, is that you are not looking for a partner or a lifelong

(4) Berkman, L. F. and Syme, S. L., *Social Networks, Host Resistance and Mortality: A nine-year follow-up study of Alameda County residents*, 1979 (Am J Epidemiol 109: 186–204)

(5) Cohen, S., Doyle, W.J., Skoner, D. P., *et al.*, *Social Ties and Susceptibility to the Common Cold*, 1997 (*Journal of the American Medical Association* 277: 1940–44)]

(6) Willcox, Bradley MD, Willcox, Craig PhD and Suzuki, Makoto MD, *The Okinawa Way* 2001, Mermaid Books

commitment. You aren't looking for a soulmate or even a new best friend. You're looking for a companion – another mum like you. Be prepared to be friends with unlikely people that at first glance you may have little in common with. Your children and your life as mums are your common bonds.

> There are about 600,000 new babies born every year in the UK. That means almost 4,000 children in your borough the same age as your child. That's 4,000 mums. Our research shows 60 per cent of mums are looking for new friends, so that's 2,400 mums looking for new friends in your area alone.

Tips for making friends

- ◆ Remember that no one will come knocking on your door; you have to get out there where the mums are.
- ◆ If you are at home with a baby or young children, make it a rule to get out of the house every day.
- ◆ Plan your week in advance. You might not need an electronic personal organiser, but you do need a little diary. Try to have something arranged for four out of five days.
- ◆ Visit a few group or class venues: you'll soon find the ones that suit you. Don't give up on any straight away. Make it a rule to persevere for three or four visits before you give up any group.
- ◆ Go to groups regularly. Week one you're a new face. Week two you know where the loos are. Week three you recognise some faces and they recognise yours. Week four you're a regular! Watch out for those new mums arriving looking lost and anxious. Can you make *them* feel welcome?
- ◆ If you work part time, make a point of doing something sociable

with your child when you're not working – even if you get to just one toddler group or activity each week. Try to prioritise this above the housework.

◆ If you work full time, you can feel excluded from the world of mums and toddlers, but remember that working mums are in the majority. There are often Saturday morning toddler groups run especially for working mums. Each one has been started by a working mum who felt she needed to meet other mums and get to know some of her child's friends. If there isn't such a group in your area, could you think about starting one?

◆ Be prepared to make the first move. It can be hard at first but with a little practice it gets easier. Look for mums who are on their own with their children. They are almost certainly as bored as you and in need of a little adult company. Open a conversation with a mum at the park or the coffee shop or the nursery.

◆ Talk to people. Talk to everyone: mums, old people, shopkeepers, neighbours. It's all good practice and it all helps to make you feel more connected to your local community. Start a conversation (see 'Conversation openers' opposite).

◆ Can you help out at the group? Do they need help making the coffee or tidying up at the end? It's all part of feeling one of the group – being on the inside – rather than on the outside looking in.

◆ Close the deal! If you feel you and the mum you've been chatting to are getting along and have something in common, don't just say goodbye – try to agree a next step. Is she coming next week? Would she like to try that Thursday group with you? How about suggesting exchanging phone numbers, so that if you are both at a loose end you could arrange to meet up? Would she and her little one like to come to your child's birthday party on Saturday?

Conversation openers

No one can resist a compliment about her child and you can always find something special to say about every child. Almost everyone likes to be asked for their advice too. Try some of these conversation openers:

- Smile and say 'Hello' to anyone and everyone. It gets easier with practice.
- 'Gorgeous baby . . . what amazing hair/eyes.'
- 'How old is your baby/child/little one?'
- 'What is his/her name? I'm Sally, by the way.'
- 'Is he/she your first?'
- 'Have you been coming here long?'
- 'Do you come here often?' (See? Just like the dating game!)
- 'Where else do you go?'
- 'Does your little one go to pre-school yet?'
- 'What school do/will your children go to?'
- 'Where do you go on rainy days?'
- 'Do you go to any (other) groups? Would you recommend it? Is there a waiting list?'
- 'Our children seem to be getting along really well. Shall we meet up again next week so they can play?'

Where do you find mums? Where do they hang out?

Start when you're pregnant

Start early to join in this mums' world – ideally, while you are pregnant. (Even if you missed this bit the first time round you can do it with your second or even third babies, so it's still relevant.) Making friends with mums and their bumps is the best preparation for parenthood you can do. Take your pick from antenatal classes, parenting classes, active birth classes, antenatal exercise classes, swimming classes and yoga classes. The friends you make will be your lifeline through late pregnancy and early motherhood. And those bumps will be your baby's first friends. Use your pregnancy to make new local friendships with other mums or mums-to-be. These are the same mums you will meet at the baby clinic for the babies' six-week check, weigh-ins and first injections, and you'll see them around town at toddler groups, at the supermarket or in the park.

It's also really good for the dads to know other dads, and friendships from antenatal classes can be powerful and long lasting. Many people use these friends to build their new social life as dinner parties and posh restaurants give way to chaotic evenings with a takeaway, a few bottles of wine and three or four tiny babies in car seats on or under the dinner table!

Where to go with baby in tow

Before you have children, you probably only see your area before nine and after five, Monday to Friday. And then you are only interested in the route to the train station, the local cinema, the decent restaurant, the takeaway and the DVD rental shop. There is a parallel universe existing in the area where you live. While the working world goes about its 'very important business', mums carry on the job of raising the next generation. Our world consists primarily of the Day People.

The Day People fall into two categories: the retired, unemployed or shift workers going about their business and mums (and grandparents and childminders) pushing prams and buggies loaded with babies and toddlers and shopping and changing bags. Before you had your baby, you might have caught a glimpse of this universe but you wouldn't have been part of it: it's not really open to non-parents. Your baby is your ticket, your free pass into a whole new world.

This next section is devoted to giving you a bit of a window into this new world, and outlining some possible entry points for you and your little one(s).

New baby groups (0–6 months)

Every mum has a health visitor assigned to them, and most health visitors will run a post-natal group of some kind. It may be a group meeting, where you can sit and chat with other new mums from the area, with the health visitor on hand to answer any questions about feeding and sleeping and so on while weighing your baby. Sadly, health visitors are having more and more families assigned to them and managing a heavier workload, so in some areas these baby groups are being replaced by weigh-in clinics that are a bit more like a visit to your doctor – you turn up, wait your turn, get your five minutes and go. Do ask your health visitor if she is running a group and where and when it is.

If there is a group, make a big effort to attend. It can be hard when your baby is very little, and sometimes the group clashes with nap time or feeding time, but it is reassuring to spend time with other mums and babies and it is a good chance to meet other new mums who live quite close. Sometimes, if a new mum is struggling, these groups can feel a bit overwhelming: the other mums all look like they've had a good night's sleep and they are laughing and smiling and generally acting as if they've got the hang of this whole baby thing. Please remember that no one finds it that easy. Ask any mums with older children how they felt during those first six months and they will all tell you the same thing: it was hard.

> **If your health visitor doesn't run a new baby group, the National Childbirth Trust (NCT) runs new parent groups specifically for first-time mums, and they also offer breastfeeding and other support. If you didn't do the NCT antenatal classes, that shouldn't stop you from joining in after the baby is born.**

Toddler groups

There are about 10,000 toddler groups meeting up each week around the country in all sorts of funny little venues. Many take place in church halls, community centres, leisure centres or that Portakabin you've never really noticed before. Before we had children, many (most?) of us were guilty of feeling superior to the mums who went to toddler groups. Sitting around a church hall with a bunch of other mums with heaps of noisy kids and instant coffee, singing 'The Wheels on the Bus'? 'Huh, not me,' we thought. 'I'll be a yummy mummy with a gorgeous baby in designer clothes chatting with friends in Starbucks!' we thought. How reality strikes. And the beauty of it is that it strikes all of us: lawyers, secretaries, waitresses, doctors, office workers, students – we were all something 'before' and now, well, we are still something and we will be something again. But right now, on this wet Tuesday morning, we are primarily mums, with babies or children to entertain and a desperate need for something to do and somewhere to go and someone to talk to! So most of us end up at the local toddler groups. Children are a great leveller. Whatever your background, income, education, size of house, skin colour or clothes size, you will have something in common with the other mums at these groups.

Contrary to general opinion and to their very name, almost every toddler group welcomes mums with new babies. Most have a baby corner with bouncy baby chairs, rugs and cushions so mums with new babies can sit and chat with somewhere comfy and safe to put their babies. So don't do what so many mums have done before and stay at home until your baby can walk!

Some of the very busy groups have waiting lists, but most don't. If you've got a phone number, give a quick call to ask if you can come along, and if you are a bit shy or nervous tell the organiser so that she can give you a bit of moral support. The organisers are usually mums themselves who will well remember being in your shoes. You often pay a small admission fee, generally 50p to £1. There are toys for the kids, coffee and usually biscuits for the mums, and often a singsong of favourite nursery rhymes at the end.

Even very young children get bored with the same setting at home. It is amazing how a grizzly child turns into a happy, sweet child when you give them a change of scene. Groups are a great way of meeting other mums with children your child's age. You will find other mums generally very friendly, but everyone agrees it can be hugely daunting the first couple of times.

If you are shy about going, try to make yourself go anyway. You don't have to talk to anyone – you won't look out of place if you don't know anyone – just go and sit in the corner and let your child sit with you or go and explore and make friends. It will get easier for you after the first few times. Remember, everyone is in the same boat with nothing better to do that day. Go to a few of these groups to start with and you will soon find the one or two where you feel most comfortable.

Swimming groups

Swimming is such a wonderful bonding activity to do with your baby. While you can happily make this an outing just for you and your child, there are also heaps of baby and toddler swimming groups where you can make new friends. The fact that you are all semi-naked and exposed in the water is great for breaking down barriers, and seeing the little ones enjoying the water makes everybody smile.

> **Most babies have a natural love of being in water, having spent nine months in fluid in the womb. Babies can be taken swimming from a very early age. Contrary to popular belief, you do not have to wait until your baby has finished his immunisation injections; you can go as soon as you both feel ready.**

The water temperature is key. You can phone ahead and ask the pool temperature. Ideally it shouldn't be less than 30 degrees, but it's unlikely that a baby swimming group would operate in a too-cold pool anyway.

Soft play

This is another one of those things you might not have come across before children – big indoor rooms full of soft squishy shapes, slides and balls for children to climb on, over and in, the idea being that they can crawl, toddle, roll or run about without danger. They can use up some of their seemingly endless energy supply while also getting great exercise to build up those little muscles. And the mums get to sit in a corner, for a while at least, and have a coffee and chat. Again, you can go alone, but try to avoid after-school hours and weekends when big kids go, as it can get a bit hectic. Better still, find out which mornings they do special mum and toddler sessions. These are often at a special price with coffee included and, more to the point, there will be more mums with younger children, many of them on their own and pleased to have someone to chat to.

Baby and toddler classes

Gym classes, music classes, art classes, dance classes – all of these are big news for our little ones. Many classes are subdivided by age: say, six months to walking, walking to two years, or two to three years. It's quite incredible how many of these little classes there are. Some are franchised, some are individual local groups, and almost all of them are run by local mums. The advantage is that most classes ask you to sign up to a term or a certain number of weeks, so you will see the same faces there each week. If you are a bit shy for toddler groups or if starting a conversation is difficult for you, you'll find this easier as it is an organised activity. You aren't left to sink or swim. And there is usually a coffee break or a chance to chat to other mums.

The park

When all else fails, get the little one in the pram or buggy and hit the park. No matter how urban your area is you are probably within walking distance of a local park. If you live in the country, there are probably prettier walks and places to amble with the buggy than the park, but the park is where the people are! The walk there is great for your figure and good for your health. Find the toddler area and hang out. Bring a flask of coffee and a packet of biscuits (to counteract any good the walk did you!) and a drink for the baby or children.

There are almost always other mums hanging about in the park with their little ones – look out for the ones on their own. Most will be delighted to engage in a bit of adult conversation.

Ask yourself:

Are you nervous or shy about meeting other mums? Are you avoiding situations where you could make new friends because of that?

1. Choose an affirmation for yourself, something like: 'I am a kind and friendly person.' Say this to yourself fifty times each morning and night. It helps it to sink into your subconscious.
2. Before you go to a group or activity, spend five minutes sitting quietly, relaxing and breathing deeply. Imagine yourself feeling confident and smiling and chatting to other mums.
3. Wear something that makes you feel good: your boots with a bit of a heel, a top you save for best, a favourite piece of jewellery that means something to you.
4. Promise yourself a treat when you get home – maybe a new magazine or a nice lunch. Your little one will have had a fun and tiring morning and may be happy to have a sleep or watch TV while you have a break.
5. Lastly, remember that if you make an effort and get a cool response from another mum in return, put it down to experience. She's probably having a bad day herself. Pick yourself up and try again with someone different.

Ask the Netmums:

Where or how did you make friends with other mums?

I met up with a couple of mums through the online Meet a Mum board on Netmums. We met for tea or coffee and chatted and now arrange meet-ups at least every week. We've even managed to get a couple of new mums to join us. We tend to chat, mooch round the shops, go to the park, go swimming sometimes . . . that kind of thing. My advice for shy mums? Don't be afraid to meet with other mums. If you find you don't like them, then don't meet with them again – but you're likely to find that you will like them.
Louisa, Southeast London, mum to Inara, 8 months

I trawled the toddler groups but never really felt part of any. I then enrolled in a baby music class. After a few weeks we all felt part of a group and gradually I built up a small group of friends. I had to visit many places before finding one where I was happy though, and it did take a lot of confidence that I sometimes didn't feel I had. My baby did enjoy the music group but she was actually very young and the chat afterwards was more important for the mums. I still meet up with three friends from this group five years down the line. We have mums' meals out without the kids every month as well as meet up for happy plays in the park en masse, and it is a lifeline.

I have surprised myself with the diverse group of friends I have – mostly through persevering in meeting up at groups and gradually getting to know people. I joined the NCT and used to hate the weekly meetings. I was about ten years younger than the other mums and felt awkward and inadequate (through no fault of theirs). I always vowed not to put myself through another coffee morning and always changed my mind and went along. One of the mums from this group is now a close friend and a vital part of my support network. She is fifteen years older than me but we found things in common and found time to talk and grew to be friends. If I had given up the groups, I would have never found this friend. For me, perseverance was the key!

Nicola, Edinburgh, mum to Hannah, 5 and Feena, 3

I got talking to a lady at the local baby massage group soon after having my daughter. She invited me out one day and that was it. We regularly get together – to play, to go out to play places or to go to the theatre – and are often on the phone or emailing, swapping experiences and asking each other questions about how our daughters are progressing. We became good friends, and we still keep in touch even though I've moved away from the area. This friendship means a lot to me, as I don't know many people where I am now. My daughter loves seeing her friend and I can see their friendship lasting a long time too. If you can get to a local group, then do it. Meeting new people gives you an opportunity to grow as a person and instills confidence in growing children.

Louise, North Staffordshire, mum to Grace, 3

Can you be at home with a gorgeous baby, have friends and family dropping in and still feel lonely? I did. At first it was more the shock of suddenly being a different person – someone's mum. I combated it by filling up every day with activity – yes, I was one of those who overstimulated their child! From about the age of three months we had music classes, swimming sessions, under-ones groups, coffee mornings, check-ups at the surgery. Then gradually we scaled it down as I made more friends and began to feel less lonely.

Then we moved house! We moved ten miles from where I grew up and thirty miles from my parents. I never thought I would have to tackle loneliness, but three months after we moved I was constantly in tears as, despite my attempts at conversation, I had met no one. I used my tactic from when I was a new mum and started seeing the same people in different places and suddenly I had a conversation starter. I met a few people from Netmums and I got in touch with the local NCT. We still have hectic days and have to plan weeks in advance, but I now have several people I can call at a moment's notice and, more importantly, people who know if they call me I will drop everything to help them. My son is three next September. How will I cope when he goes to nursery school?!
Claire, Worksop, mum to Luke, 2

I was really lucky, as we had a fairly chatty post-natal group (it was run by the clinic), and a girl I was friendly with and I decided that we should bite the bullet and invite everyone we spoke to at the group for coffee. Scary, but it worked and now three years on most of us meet up with at least four to five of the group (we were thirteen at our maximum!) on a regular basis. We started with coffee each week in a local place and then when the children were older we started going to each other's houses. It was great, as we gained a close circle of friends who all understood how we felt, and now our children have a wonderful set of friends who we hope will stay with them for a long time.

It was scary to take the plunge and ask people, but I've found that the best way to meet people when you have a baby is to take a deep breath, banish the nervous voices in your head and just say, 'Hi' to the person standing next to you. You never know where it might lead! I'd also have to say that parent and toddler groups have been a great thing for my son and me. Both of us get to meet new people, he has fun playing and I get the chance to have an 'adult' conversation!

Shelley, Bushey, mum to Callum, 3

I definitely feel that, throughout your children's lives, if you stay open to friendship and welcome talking and making approaches – just smile or say, 'Hello', etc. yourself – you do get to know more people. There are people at the school daily whom I have barely spoken to and mostly it is because they come across as so unapproachable – they never smile, they don't respond to me smiling at them, and after a while I give up trying. I do wonder if they are really as standoffish as they appear and believe they probably aren't. No matter how shy you are, at least you ought to acknowledge other people's attempts at contact, because a smile develops into a 'Hello', a 'Hello' into 'How are you?' and then it's on to proper conversation. If you can't return a smile or, even worse, look away when someone does smile at you, then people won't take it further. I used to be the shy one who looked away, kept herself huddled in the corner, avoiding any eye contact with anyone, and it was a long time before I realised I was alienating myself from everyone else. But once I smiled back, I started to find people would approach me – and come back a second time.

Sharron, Luton, mum to Louisa, 5 and Samantha, 2

Over the years I've made lots of mum-friends through toddler groups, school, etc. and I have a mixture of a couple of very close mum-friends who go back to the births of our first children thirteen years ago, and several more casual mum-friends I've met since having my subsequent three children. I am always friendly and chatty to other mums at the various baby groups I go to now, but I'm on my fourth child and have a demanding job as well. I wonder if I'm maybe seen as unfriendly by other mums sometimes when I can't always meet for coffee, etc. So I do tend to accept a lot of invitations to coffee, which then make me feel stressed because I don't really have enough time to keep them! I'd rather this than hurt people's feelings though. I always think when someone says, 'Do you want to get together for coffee?' that it might have taken them lots of courage to ask, so I can't bear to say, 'No.' I'd rather be stressed! Sometimes I ask if we can make it in a few weeks' time, but I rarely refuse outright. I remember the first time I walked into a toddler group thirteen years ago and a few (not all) of the mums just ignored me. I've always sworn I'll not be like that and I'm not!

Sue, Leeds, mum of three boys and a girl

When I just had my daughter I was suffering from really bad post-natal depression. My husband was working full time and I was a new mum alone with hardly any family around to ask for advice or help. Most of my friends didn't have children and therefore didn't want to know me or help either. It got to the point where I would fake being ill so that my husband would stay at home and I would have him for company all day. Family rarely visited and as a new mum it was daunting looking after this little person.

Just when I thought it couldn't get any worse, my community midwife and community psychiatric nurse told me about my local Sure Start. They offered a mother and baby group for new mums and mums-to-be. They also offered all sorts of courses, etc. for people in my area. I joined straight away and went to the groups. I made some really good friends who were in the same position as me, understood me and helped me with advice and support. These friends are now my main contacts for support and we meet up and have a chat every week. I also found Netmums shortly after and have made some really good friends there too. I wish I had known about it sooner! I guess I'd just say that even though you think there is no support for you, there is; you just have to look and ask around. If it wasn't for Sure Start and Netmums, I certainly would be a very lonely mummy!

Cheryl, Rotherham, mum to Amber, 2

I have made some email friends through Netmums and even found a girl I went to school with. Any new mums I would advise to browse the Meet a Mum section and reply to anyone who sounds like you.

Jacqui, Peterborough, mum to Liam, 7, Zack, 5 and Ellis, 10 months

I worked full time all my life until I had a baby at thirty-seven. None of my friends had children and my social life disappeared overnight. A toddler group saved my sanity.

The one nearest the children's school, so that you then know someone at the school gates, is best. I took my ten-week-old baby and, although there was not much in it for him at the time, I was made very welcome. My son is ten years old now and still plays with the children he went to toddlers with. I also keep in touch with the mums.
Sylvia, North Hants, mum to Alex, 10 and Joe, 8

When I first gave up work to look after my daughter, I did not know any other mums in the area who were also at home. My daughter and I joined a Jo Jingles class [see p. 311] and it was great to see like-minded people and their children. It took a few months, but after each class I got chatting to other mums and eventually suggested a couple of us get together for coffee. The children then played or we organised days out. I have now made two great friends this way and we have had some lovely days out. The children love playing together and it means I can have some adult chat too. It's great, as we can swap tips, share any worries, etc. I now no longer feel isolated. This has given me the confidence to chat to anyone now when I go to activities with my daughter and to make new friends.
Kelly, Leicestershire, mum to Daisy, 2

When I had my first child, I was living in a very quiet area. My family live about a hundred miles away and my only friends were through work. I was so lonely I used to walk to the nearest supermarket every day just to have a coffee. Luckily, we moved to a livelier area when my son was four months old. The health visitors ran a weekly New Parent group for three months. It was a godsend. Not only did I get lots of invaluable advice but I also made a circle of friends that is still going strong two years (and more babies) later. I really feel that more health visitors should be encouraged to arrange similar groups. Also, I resolved *never* knowingly to leave another mum feeling lonely and isolated, so I go out of my way to welcome new mums at any group I go to. We are all in the same boat, so let's help each other out. P.S. I now have more friends than I've ever had in my life!

Debra, Rotherham, mum to Finn, 2 and Louis, 8 months

My breakthrough came when I met someone from Netmums. We really connected and she introduced me to other people she knew. Together we joined the National Childbirth Trust [see p. 318] and we now help to run groups encouraging mums to meet and chat and form friendships, as well as offering antenatal classes and breastfeeding counselling.

My advice to anyone expecting, or in a similar situation to the one I was in, is to join the NCT or at least go along to some of their events (you don't have to be a member). It's run by parents for parents and you should get a warm welcome!

Loraine, Nottingham, mum to Sam, 3

2 Children Behaving Badly

Do you ever look at your children and wonder where you are going wrong? Do they whinge and whine, argue and fight all day? Constantly *want* everything? Throw things? Hit out? Embarrass you in public? Let you down in front of your family and friends? Welcome to the world of parenting. Please take a moment here to reassure yourself that what you are experiencing is completely normal and is something every other parent is going through, has been through or is going to go through.

We don't give birth and suddenly find ourselves equipped with the tools of good parenting. Frankly, unless you have a PhD in child psychology, it's nearly impossible to know how best to react to your toddler screaming the supermarket down because he wants to open the egg-box and play with the eggs. Even if you read all the parenting manuals and it all seems to make perfect sense on paper, somehow your child will find a way to beat the system. Just when you are practising your calm and controlled techniques, they find a way to push you over the edge. They seem to know exactly what button to press, and if they press that button as your boss phones, you tip the milk bottle over and the pizza starts burning, and you may react in a way quite different from that advised in the childcare manual!

What is good parenting?

Good parenting is not about ironing all the laundry, including vests and socks, zapping every germ from every surface, having floors you can eat off and washing the net curtains every week. It is not about having a perfectly ordered house, a freezer full of home-made dinners, and a policy of not leaving the table until you have eaten everything on your plate. It is not about having a strict routine with a bath and hair wash every night at 6.30pm with no exceptions and everyone up and dressed by 7am. It is not about having children who can read by the time they are three, know all their times tables by the time they start school and are on the professional tennis circuit by the time they are eight, guaranteeing a scholarship to a good school.

Good parenting is about having a collectively happy home: not a home where the parents are happy but the children are seen and not heard nor a home where the children happily run wild but the parents are run ragged. It's about finding a balance so that everyone has a chance to do their thing. It's about sharing and it's about rights. One person's rights end when they start to infringe on someone else's rights. Your child sometimes needs to be noisy and play loud games but not when the baby is settling to sleep. Your child has a right to tell you that he is full and doesn't want to eat any more but not to have pudding instead of his dinner after you've cooked for him. You have the right to put your feet up and expect the children to play alone while you read the paper but perhaps for twenty minutes not for three hours (if only!). Children have a right to have toys and lay them out and play with them but you have a right to relax in the evening in a home that isn't littered with toys that haven't been put away. And so on.

The whole thing is a balancing act. If you can remember that, rather than trying to ensure it's always the children who are happy, it gets easier. You start to see the trade-offs. And you start to keep a mental balance sheet. It's also good for your children to know that life isn't all about them. There are other people and their rights matter.

What is so wrong with good old-fashioned discipline?

A child needs to assert himself, to learn to express his opinions and preferences and to learn to make his own decisions. If parents overpower a child every time and use physical (or emotional) *force* through their power as adults to get the child to do as he is told, the child will learn to react in one of two ways: he'll give up and relinquish his power – he'll become submissive and unwilling or even incapable of asserting himself and of arguing his own case or standing up for himself; or he'll hold all his little losses inside – all those times he felt overcome and powerless will be stored up and can one day turn to anger and rebellion. This might manifest in his relationships with other children (the bullied becomes the bully) or in his behaviour at home either now or in the future as he begins to rebel.

Try not to think in terms of winners and losers. One of the keys to creating a happy atmosphere at home is to banish the idea that if your child gets his own way, he wins and you lose, or if you get him to do what you want, you win and he loses. The idea of winners and losers immediately implies that your home is a battleground and that's exactly what we are trying to avoid. Good parenting is often about compromise, about balance and about creating a win–win solution. It can seem like a bit (or a lot) of extra effort but, as with all things in life, a little effort goes a long way and the pay-off of a happy home in which conflict is reduced is a tremendous reward.

Setting the scene

Babies and children are incredibly sensitive to mood and atmosphere. Before you try to mould or change your children's behaviour, look at your own. Are you, without realising it, saying to your child, 'Do as I say, not as I do'? Your children are often like little mirrors held up to your emotions and your behaviour.

Ask yourself:

Is my own behaviour influencing my children's behaviour?

Can you spend a couple of days watching yourself, observing your actions and behaviour? Perhaps by asking yourself some of these questions you can see how their behaviour may actually be related to your own.

◆ What is the atmosphere like in your home?
Is it frenetic, with everyone rushing about, needing to be somewhere on time? Are you constantly 'doing jobs' and rarely sitting down with a magazine? Do you expect them to be calm when you never are? Maybe it's the opposite: is it a lethargic sort of atmosphere? No one likes getting out of bed and then no one likes getting dressed and everyone spends as long as possible on the sofa?

◆ How are you feeling inside?
What are your main emotions: frustration, resentment, boredom? Can you find any sign of contentment, joy, peace? Are you an openly emotional person? Or do you keep your feelings hidden? Do you cry in front of the children and tell them when you are feeling sad? Do you talk about feelings – both yours and theirs – with your children?

◆ How do you interact with other people?
Are you asking your children to play nicely when you've spent hours arguing in front of them with your mother-in-law, your ex-best friend, the shop manager and even the milkman? Do you expect them to speak in a normal voice when everyone else shouts? Try imagining your conversations through the eyes of your child. What are they seeing and what are they hearing?

◆ How about you and their dad?
How do you get on? Are you nice to each other? Do you chat to each other or bark instructions and argue about who had the hardest day? If you argue with each other, do you make up in front of the children to illustrate the fact that you might not always agree but you can go on loving

each other? Do you do little things for each other like bringing up a cup of tea in the morning? Do you have any shared interests or things you do together as a family? Or do you tend to take it in turns to entertain the children? Do you agree with each other's ideas on parenting and back each other up? Can you and he spend a bit of time discussing some of the specific aspects of parenting that cause you stress and that you have different views on? Discuss issues such as bedtimes and meal times, and agree how you can deal with them. This is harder than it sounds, as you have both been brought up differently and will have different ideas of what constitutes 'good parenting'. It needs careful negotiation between you. Even if you are separated from the children's father, it is important for children to have a consistent approach from both parents. If not, they end up confused and will play you off against each other, which will lead to more conflict.

◆ And you and them?
  How much time do you spend with each child each day, just one on one? How much eye contact do you have with your child? Do you listen to them? (Really listen?) How do you ask your children to do something (like get their shoes and coat on)? And what do you do if they don't do it?

Positive parenting techniques

Try adopting some of these very simple positive parenting techniques:

Engage
Listen to your children, really listen . . . If they are talking to you,

rather than keeping your back to them while you wash up or browse the internet, stop, kneel down to their level, look them in the eye and listen to what they are saying. When the children argue and fight, instead of shouting them down, listen to their points of view.

Whether you're at work most of the day or spending all your time with your children, can you take twenty minutes to focus on them and no one else? Can you be with them, in the moment and not half-heartedly, thinking about all the chores that need doing or stuff that you'd rather be doing? Whether you have a young baby or an older child, find something to do that they will appreciate. Sing them nursery rhymes, build a great Lego creation together, play dolls, bake a cake, read to them and talk to them about the story, or do an art or craft activity. Let them choose an activity you can do together and don't take over.

Be patient

If you want to know what is going on in your child's life and what is on his mind, then don't try the direct approach. Don't fire questions at him, such as: 'What did you do at school?' 'Who did you play with?' 'How was your day?' Children always seem to do 'nothing much' at school, play with 'no one' and their day was 'OK'.

In fact, the time when you are most likely to find out about your child and what's going on in his mind is when you are quietly working on an activity side by side or snuggling on the bed together at bedtime. When you are just spending time together, busy doing nothing, you'll get those golden snippets, such as 'I hate Johnny 'cos he always pushes me.'

Praise and encourage

Catch your child doing something right rather than doing something wrong. Try it. You might have to look hard at first but praise and attention for positive behaviour leads to more good behaviour. Don't sum it all up by saying, 'You were very good today.' Instead, praise the little things: 'That's lovely to see you sitting at the table', 'That was very good sharing. I'm proud of you', 'Did you put your own socks/coat/shoes on? That's very clever of you.'

Accept
Your child is a special and wonderful little person. He is also unique, so don't try to compare him with other children. If he's scared of balloons, or won't shake hands with Mickey Mouse at Disneyland, respect that. Never ridicule or use sarcasm on your child. Don't try to mould him into being something he isn't. Create an atmosphere of acceptance in the house. Children have to make mistakes in order to learn. Praise their efforts rather than criticise their failures.

Let the little things go
If you come down heavily on your child every time something is spilt or broken, or every time he steps out of line, or each time something he does annoys you, then you'll always be on at the poor child. Children are clumsy and messy and noisy. Even when they mean to be good or want to be good, they often forget the rules. Try to let the little things go. That way you can work more effectively on the bigger stuff.

Show love
You are the centre of your child's world. You are the most important person, place or thing in his world. Remember most of his behaviour, good or bad, is calculated to get *your* attention in some form or other. Show him how important he is to you. As well as kisses goodnight and kisses goodbye, show him lots of other demonstrations of love. You know your child best, so think about what means most to him or her. If your child is a cuddly child, give loads of extra cuddles and hugs. Swoop on him when he's playing

and least expecting it and say, 'Oooh, I just had to come and kiss you', or call him to you for a cuddle rather than waiting for him to ask for one. Ruffle his hair as he walks past; hold his hand in the garden or when you're watching TV together. Other children might prefer a less physical show of love but would like to know that you are watching them while they play, or have you join their game or just sit companionably beside them with your book rather than in a different room. Maybe you could have a secret signal, like a hand squeeze, that he can use to mean 'I'm feeling a bit sad or worried.'

As often as possible, spend ten minutes with your child at bedtime. After his story, just before or just after lights out, sit there quietly for those minutes while he gets into a relaxed and pre-sleep state. This is the moment that things will pass through his head and if you're there he might tell you about them. It's a great time to share his worries and reassure him before sleep.

Have fun

Children love absolutely nothing more than seeing their parents having a laugh and a joke with them. It makes them feel the world is perfect. You are down at their level, you are connecting with them, you are pleased with them and you are happy. Remember a lot of bad behaviour is an effort to get your attention. If you are having fun with your child, there is no need for him to act badly.

Beware of labelling your child

It is hugely tempting to try to classify your children according to their personality. It can become a self-fulfilling prophecy. Be careful that you don't label your child 'the difficult one', 'the fat one', 'the stupid one' or 'the lazy one'. Children, with their beautiful simplicity, will believe what you tell them and show you how it is true. They will do what they believe you expect of them. Positive praise has a positive effect, but try to use praise specifically. Tell your child how helpful he was at the shops, or how kind he was sharing his toys, or how tidy he was folding his pyjamas.

Also, brothers or sisters of 'the good one' will automatically know that this means they are 'the naughty ones'. Watch your behaviour and your language for signs of labelling, and be especially careful when talking to other adults about your children – they hear everything! Even if your child is busily playing and it seems as if he isn't listening, children have an amazing ability to absorb the content of conversations.

Getting your child to carry out an instruction

To avoid getting to the 'Right, *that's it*! I've asked you three times to put your shoes on, no more TV for the rest of your life' stage, try some of these techniques for getting your child to do what needs to be done.

1. Give clear, calm instructions
When you want your child to do something, try not to bellow it across the room while you are doing something else. Stop what you are doing, go over and kneel in front of your child and make eye contact. Calmly and clearly explain what you want and why. 'Please get your shoes and put them on, as we need to leave.'

2. Give a time warning
It is more respectful of your children and therefore more effective if you try to give a time warning that they must shortly finish their game or leave what they are doing. 'In five minutes you are going to have to leave, so it's time to finish your game.' Think how you would feel if you were in the middle of something and had to drop it immediately.

3. Avoid system overload

'Finish your breakfast, brush your teeth, get your shoes and coat on and get your bags.' By the time he has finished his breakfast, he'll be distracted and have forgotten everything else!

4. Try making it into a game

Few children can resist games. 'Let's see if you can put your shoes on before I count to ten.' 'Let's see if you can put your shoes on before I finish my washing up.' 'Can you keep your hands in the air the whole time I'm putting your shoes on?' Using a teddy bear or glove puppet to initiate the games can work magic. For instance, Teddy says, 'Can you show me how you eat your breakfast? Oooh, you're good at that. Show me again. Can I have some?'

5. Offer an alternative

Sometimes let your child make choices – simple choices. 'Do you want to wear your trainers or wellies?' If she doesn't respond, try choosing the one you know she likes least: 'Mmm, OK, I'll choose – trainers, I think.' You've got to be happy with the choice, so be careful what you offer. For example, if you really want her to choose the wellies, as it is tipping down with rain outside, don't offer trainers if you're worried about wet feet and ruined shoes. If you offer the choice, you have to be able to live with the consequences of the decision!

> You can also cleverly use it to turn a chore into a game. Try putting their shoes on their ears or their hands. Ask them: 'I can't seem to remember where these shoes go on. Can you remember?' Or 'Do you know how these shoes do up? I can't do it.'

6. Let them show off

Children love to demonstrate their skills and their ability to solve problems. They particularly adore the role-swap of showing mum, dad or a grandparent how something should be done or doing something better than you. You can use this in games time and time again: when building blocks, let yours fall over while theirs stays straight and tall; in a race to the gate they will giggle in delight at beating you.

7. Counting to three

Having asked once or twice to no avail, say, in a calm voice, 'I want those shoes on before I get to three. Onnnnnnne, Twooooooooooo, Two and a haaaaaaaaalf, Thr . . .' The idea is that you don't actually ever get to three. Many mums of children from about two up to twleve (or more) find this good old counting to three technique works every time. While you are counting, your child still has control over the situation. Your child is making the decision, whether to put the shoes on or not, whether to comply with you and get your approval or go against you. This is very powerful, as none of us – not even little children – likes feeling a loss of control and having our decision-making powers taken away from us. If you do get to three, they have chosen *not* to comply and you get to take over. Show that you are in charge now: quickly scoop up the child and put him in the car or buggy (even without shoes).

Ask yourself:

What can I learn from something bad happening?

Each time a situation gets out of hand, review this ABC.

Antecedents: What led up to this happening? Were we all rushed? Was the baby screaming and affecting the older children? Was my mind elsewhere?

Behaviour: How did they and I behave or what did we do? For instance, I shouted at them, they responded by shouting back, and then they shouted at each other.

Consequences: What was the outcome? They all ended up in tears, I was even more stressed and we were late anyway.

This way you can learn from your experiences. Also try using the ABC when something GOOD happens – when you have one of those lovely family moments when everything seems right. Can you learn from that too and introduce the same elements a bit more often?

Your flashpoints

We've talked about letting the little things go, but what are the big things? Rather than trying to change everything about your child's behaviour in one go, can you think about what really drives you mad? What is your key flashpoint?

- It might be that the kids try to hang around all evening rather than go to bed at a specific time, so you don't get the couple of hours of grown-up time that you really need.
- Is it that you work so hard keeping the house tidy and everyone else throws stuff around and no one else picks anything up?
- Do you cook lovely dinners every day only for them to go uneaten by ungrateful children?
- Is it the constant whinging?

- Maybe you hate shopping as it's always so stressful and it always ends up in a screaming scene at the checkout?

What matters most to you might not seem important to another family, hence the need to 'personalise' your children's behaviour. Many families don't mind having the children around in the evenings, so everyone muddles along until they feel ready for bed. But if you are desperate for some space by 8pm, you'll find your feelings getting increasingly out of control and you'll lose your ability to be calm and rational. In turn, the children pick up on this and play up even more until a full-scale Stonehenge-sized vicious circle is set up.

The 80/20 rule probably applies to you here: 20 per cent of the behaviour is causing 80 per cent of your stress and unhappiness. If you can identify your flashpoint, then you can put a plan together to deal with it.

Ask yourself:

Which behavioural issue would you most like to change in your child? What is the one thing that causes you most stress?

If you have a partner, discuss it together. Is it the same one?

Make it SMART:

Specific: What exactly is the issue? *My child won't go to bed so I don't get any me-time in the evenings.*

Measurable: What would be a good outcome? *My child would be in bed by 7.30pm even if she's not asleep.*

Achievable: Is that possible? *Yes (depending on the age of the child and the time she gets up).*

Realistic: Is it realistic to expect this outcome given the way your lives are at present? *Well, I don't get in from work until 7 and she is so excited to see me that she won't go to bed so perhaps it isn't realistic to expect her to let go of me so quickly. Maybe I need to rethink the bedtime to 8pm so I can spend an extra half an hour reading to her.*

Timely: When are you going to start? *We've got friends coming tomorrow so the evening after that.*

And then add on an EA:

Explicit: Explain to your child what will happen from now on and what's expected. *'When the clock gets to here (show 7.30pm) Mummy will snuggle down with you and read you a story until the clock gets to here (show 8pm) and then we'll turn the light off and put your music on and Mummy will go and have her dinner and you'll settle down to sleep.'*

Agreed: Get your child to agree.
Does that sound OK to you? Are we going to do that? And you won't get out of bed after the story?

Five steps to changing a specific behaviour pattern

(Suitable from age two upwards)

1. Decide what behaviour you are trying to change and a reasonable target to achieve: 'I want my child to stop using that whining voice for everything.' 'I want my child not to leave the table at teatime.'
2. Have a very formal family meeting. Set it up around the table, with paper and pens. Get the whole family involved (even if that means just you and your two year old). Explain that this particular behaviour is unacceptable because . . . Tell them because of that, from right now, it isn't to happen again. Write down the aim for the family and ask everyone to sign it, even the little ones.
3. Agree the process: 'If you whine when you want something, I won't be able to get it for you and we'll have to wait until you ask nicely.' 'When I say that tea is ready, you will sit at your place until you've finished your meal and then ask to get down.'
4. Agree the reward: 'If you manage to sit at the table nicely and ask to get down when you've finished, then you will get a sticker on your chart or a small prize.' (see Rewards, below)
5. Get them to buy in. Ask your child if he understands, then write it all on a Post-it and stick it on the fridge. You can then constantly refer to it: 'Do you remember?'

Serious stuff

You also need to decide what behaviour is not acceptable for your children. This might include hitting, swearing, being rude to adults, going out of the garden gate or crossing a road without you. Once you have decided what is not acceptable, be very clear. There are no exceptions to this particular behaviour and no excuses – even if it's the holidays, or they are tired, or they've been through a rough time lately.

> If your child is doing something really naughty or dangerous, go straight to the point: get down to her level, look her in the eye and speak in a very serious, calm voice. 'You must not hit your sister. It is unacceptable behaviour. Do you understand?'

This is the non-negotiable behaviour, the line that cannot be crossed. You shouldn't even need to have a sanction – it is simply a NO. Try to take some time to think about why your child might be behaving in this way. Try to think it through from her point of view. Is she trying to get your attention to keep you busy with her? Is she seeking revenge and trying to get even with you? Are you having a power battle with your child about who is in control? Is the child trying to show you that she needs you? If you know why your child is behaving in a certain way, then it is easier to see how you might manage that behaviour.

Rewards

Rewards can be a very useful positive parenting technique and there are a few ways to get the best out of them. Used in isolation, they aren't really rewards at all but bribes and that can be fine – as long as you recognise that. The danger is that good behaviour becomes something unusual to be rewarded rather than something that is an everyday part of life.

It's helpful to put rewards in the context of adult life. How many of us would go to work for no salary? And yet, it has been shown time and again that money is not the prime motivator of a workforce. Recognition, feeling important and valued, being part of the decision-making – without such things in a work place the staff may still do the bare minimum to get through the day, and they'll still get paid, but they'll be pretty miserable and, as soon as they get the chance, they'll be out of there. Can you relate that to your child? Before offering rewards (or bribes) re-read the section on positive parenting techniques (see pp. 47–50) to make sure you've got the framework in place.

Make a sticker chart with the children's help and decide the reward. The best rewards are perhaps those that involve the whole family. So when eight stickers (or ten or whatever) have been awarded, the whole family does something fun: pizzas and a DVD, or a trip to soft play or the cinema. Let your child choose what she would like to do. Alternatively, for something more immediate, have a reward bag or box filled with small but fun items (if possible, wrapped up like a lucky dip). Go to the pound shop and stock up on little bits and novelty items – preferably 50p to £1's worth. Occasionally, catch your child being good (bringing his plate from the table without being asked, or staying nice and quiet while you take a long phone call), bring out your reward bag and surprise him with a prize.

Be aware of the impact a reward chart is having or may have on him. It must allow him to see that he is a success and to show others that he is a success – an empty star chart is a sign of failure. Likewise, a star chart where a sibling is flying ahead with stars while he is still on the starting block is not going to feel motivating, but it will feel like failure, so don't pit siblings against each other.

The principles of using star charts or stickers

1. Only use them from about the age of three, when children can begin to understand the concept.
2. Keep star charts as a way of helping to change a child's behaviour and target only one or maybe two behaviours at a time so your child isn't confused and overwhelmed.
3. Involve your children: talk to them calmly about how it will work and make sure they understand how they earn a sticker. Make the chart together and let them choose the reward.
4. Make sure that you give the sticker/star immediately. As soon as they reach the goal, make sure they get the agreed reward as soon as possible – otherwise the child may not associate the reward with his new, better behaviour.
5. Review the chart with your children to keep them actively involved in their progress and praise their successes.
6. Never take stars or stickers or any other sort of reward away. Lack of rewards will be sufficient.

Consequences

So you've tried everything. You've tried distractions, offering alternatives, rewarding with stickers, turning it into a game – turning yourself inside out – and still you are getting a big fat NO. It's time to look at consequences. It's worth a final warning: 'This is your last chance. I'm going to count to three' and then counting quickly: 'One. Two.' If they start showing an effort, slow down your count. Otherwise, if they look defiant or are ignoring you, hit the Three.

Rather than 'punishments', try to think in terms of 'consequences'. Your child is offered choices and her choice comes with a consequence. The choice she makes will have a positive or a negative consequence; it is your child who has made that choice!

The idea is to show your child that the outcome is in her hands. It's she, not you, who made the choice and therefore it is she, not you, who has chosen the negative consequence. For example, a child might be given the choice to change out of her school uniform and play in the garden or leave her uniform on and stay inside the house. Try to remain positive in the way that you offer the choices. 'You can go out to play when you have changed your uniform' might be better than 'You can't go out until you've changed out of your uniform.'

Before the behaviour that you are finding unacceptable occurs, agree with your child what will happen if this behaviour occurs again. Try to make the consequences logical so that they follow on from the behaviour. For example, if she still goes in the garden in her uniform, she must come inside and cannot go in the garden for, say, half an hour.

Time out

Everyone has a different take on this, but fundamentally the concept involves removing the child from everyone else and putting him in a place that is quiet, boring and lonely (although never scary). The bottom step of the stairs is a common favourite. The most important thing is that it is done calmly and consistently. 'If you don't do/continue to do something, then I will put you on the bottom step. One. Two. Three.' And take him by the hand or carry him to the step. Tell him he must stay there for an agreed period of time (some experts suggest one minute for each year, i.e. a three year old should stay there for three minutes). He can get down only when you tell him he can. It can take a long time and a bit of 'putting back' the first few times but stick with it – the child will soon get the hang of it. Never overpower your child and make sure you win; get him to acknowledge and realise when his behaviour hasn't been reasonable or acceptable. When he gets off the step, maybe have a quick hug and change the subject. Start again with a clean sheet, no hard feelings – it's over.

This is not recommended as a first course of action as it is a punishment that can be quite overwhelming for the child. It should be reserved only for really serious problems, for example, hitting out at others.

The principles of time out

1. Time out isn't suitable for children under the age of three.
2. Time out should be used for only one or two clearly defined behaviours.
3. It should be planned with your child before being implemented. She should know what will happen if she acts a certain way and why.
4. You need to remain calm and not be angry or aggressive. It shouldn't feel scary for your child; it's a matter of fact, a consequence of her behaviour.
5. Put your child in time out as soon as the behaviour occurs and leave her for no longer than one minute for every year of the child's age.
6. Don't talk (or argue) with your child when placing her in time out or while she is there.
7. After she has calmed down and is behaving well, give praise and attention to how well she has calmed down.
8. Use time out consistently or your child will become confused and it won't have any beneficial effect.
9. Choose a positive behaviour to reward. For example, if time out is used for hitting out at others, then playing nicely together might be targeted as a behaviour that might be rewarded.

Planned ignoring

In a child's eyes, even negative attention is attention. By giving lots of attention to negative behaviour, you may be reinforcing it. Some unacceptable behaviour may be managed by ignoring it. This is suitable only for behaviour that does not put the child or others in danger, e.g. tantrums, swearing and squabbling.

The principles of planned ignoring

1. Plan to ignore only one or two behaviours at a time; these should be made known to your child where possible.
2. Ignored behaviour may come as a shock to your child, who may redouble his efforts to get a reaction. Be aware that he is testing you and remain consistent.
3. You might be able to continue what you are doing at the time or you might need to turn away from your child to be able to ignore the behaviour effectively. Avoid doing or saying anything to your child and do not make eye contact during the 'ignoring'.
4. Keep your child in sight so that you can respond as soon as the behaviour changes. As soon as the unacceptable behaviour ceases, give your child lots of positive attention. With an older child, it may be necessary to talk through the incident.

Crisis-coping techniques

And then there are those days when you just can't cope. You've not slept well, you've a headache and the house is a mess . . . and the kids choose today to be their absolute devil-children worst. Do they know how you are feeling? Is that why they are doing it? Do they hate you that much? It can seem that way, but it's probably because they sense that you are withdrawn from them today. They are trying to provoke a reaction from you to show them that you are still there, still mum, even if you are a cross mum.

Or it could be that they are being no worse than usual but on another day you would cope with it differently. Today is the day when you've no inner resources left – no imagination for alternatives and no energy to distract them with games or activities.

- ◆ Run a bath, even if it's the middle of the day, and all get in together.
- ◆ Drop everything and take them for a walk. The fresh air and activity will do you all good.
- ◆ Go out for tea. Even if it's a burger and chips, it means you get out of the house and don't have to cook or wash up.
- ◆ Call a friend and ask if you can all go over there. Be honest – say you're having a bad day and you'll happily repay her on her next bad day.
- ◆ Have a pyjama day: no one gets dressed, lots of DVDs and popcorn. The world won't stop if you all take a day off.
- ◆ Imagine yourself inside a bubble. Nothing out there can touch you; you are inside a big, safe, quiet plastic bubble – weird but strangely effective.

Imagine how you would describe the scene to your best friend or partner later on. Is there a funny side? It might not seem like it right now, but you might be able to see something funny about it later.

Ask the Netmums:

How do you manage your child's behaviour?

My daughter loves stickers, so I use that as a motivator to encourage her to try hard at swimming or for helping me without being asked. I praise her lots and encourage her to make decisions for herself and do things herself (fasten her coat, choose a sandwich filling). I also show her that, at times, I make the decisions and she has to do whatever has been asked (hold my hand to cross the road, eat her tea at the table). I try to make things fun. We race up to bed each night! I say, 'I'll win', she heads upstairs and I go and get the potty. We both know she's going to win, but she's laughing and giggling while getting into bed. We don't have to fight about it.

On the odd occasion when she refuses to listen or does something she knows not to, I tend to sit her away from me. It's not a naughty step as such, but with her back to me (even in the local shop on one occasion). She usually cries and then I'll go back to her and ask her why she's been sat out to show me she understands what's going on. She'll apologise and then we move on to more positive things.
Louise, North Staffordshire, mum to Grace, 3

I use a three-step 'formula'. First, I get my son's attention. I usually crouch down and get him to look at me; often an instruction such as 'Point to mummy's nose' gets him looking at me and responding. Then I talk to him in a calm way, explaining why what he is doing is not what I want him to do or not appropriate, etc. Lastly, the most important step and the one easily forgotten, I wait and allow him time to process what I've said. Sometimes the simplest of questions will take him a few seconds to respond to even when he's cooperating fully.

The thing I've found that works best to avoid getting into problems is to forewarn him all the time of what is going to happen. For example, I'll say, 'We will read this book and then put on our shoes and go out.' But you have to be consistent and do what you say. I can be quite bad about changing my mind and that really confuses him.

Irina, Ayrshire, mum to Max, 2

Give lots and lots of praise, especially when you finally get them to do something you've asked. Although it can be very hard to switch from angry 'do as you're told' mammy to happy 'well done' mammy in a matter of seconds, don't hold grudges! Cali really reacts well to praise and being told she has made me happy; her little face just lights up. The naughty step does not work for us, as I discovered today. Earlier in the week I had introduced the naughty step when Cali wasn't doing as she was told; today when I asked her to tidy up she decided the naughty step was preferable and went and sat on it of her own accord!

Rachel, Teesside, mum to Cali-Rose, 3

Try to phrase things in a positive rather than a negative way. For example, say, 'Please walk' instead of, 'Don't run.' Getting used to doing this is surprisingly difficult (or was for me) but it does pay off and I feel less 'naggy' as a mum. Also, look for the good (or, if that is not happening, the nearly good) and praise, praise, praise – even small things, such as 'You are sitting so nicely at the table' (despite him wriggling beforehand). Catch it and praise it!

After a bad bit (everyone has been awful, you have lost it and even the cat is cowering), change the mood and forgive. Put on some music, get an activity out or splash in puddles. Don't dwell on it. Deliberately try to change the mood and often you will feel happier and your children will follow. Give lots and lots of spur of the moment cuddles, tickles, strokes and 'I love yous' – all the time.
Nicola, Edinburgh, mum to Hannah, 5 and Feena, 3

Say 'sorry' when you misbehave. I have learnt that it goes a long way and they truly understand that it is OK to make mistakes. It also shows respect towards them.
Claudia, Bedford, mum to Sophia, 5 and Mia, 3

I would have to say, 'Treat them with respect and in turn they will learn to do the same.' Say when you have done something wrong and teach them to say 'sorry', 'please' and 'thanks'. Remember they learn from you every day, so act in a way you would like them to be. Also encourage their independence. Let them try new things even if you may think they are a little young. Love them and cherish them. Don't spoil them with gifts such as toys and sweets but with time spent doing things together, such as making cakes or painting.
Wendy, Northampton, mum to Caitlin, 3

Spend as much time as you can with your kids, and always be willing to talk about anything with them. This builds a great relationship with your kids, which is vital, particularly as they get older!
Sue, Leeds, mum of three boys and a girl

Well, I'll tell you how my five year old handles my misbehaviour, as sometimes we can follow the children's example. When I occasionally shout at him, he pulls a humorous face and makes me laugh. When I apologised to him for shouting at him the other day, he said, 'Oh, that's all right, Mum, as long as you say, "Sorry." Anyway, I know it's just because you're a bit stressed and you still love me and I love you too!'
Kerry, Halifax, mum to Oliver, 5 and Daisy, 17 months

For me it has to be *routine* and *promises* (not idle threats). I found out quite quickly that if you stick to the routine, no matter what, things run really smoothly and your child/children feel safe, secure and willing. I also found out quite quickly that if you make idle threats you get nowhere. If you are going to say something, make it a promise and stick to it. For instance, if your child misbehaves and you say something like, 'If you don't stop throwing your things around, I will put them in the bin', then put them in the bin, and make sure that your child sees you do it. It works absolute wonders. My children are 16, 16 and 18 now, and it still works.
Dawn, Stoke-on-Trent, mum to Rebecca, 18, Andrew, 16 and Laura, 16

Be consistent. Don't lose your temper if you can possibly help it. *Never* shout; it only makes you madder and the kids scared! (Impossible, I know, but at least try!) Try to listen and comment when toddlers are jabbering, because they are trying to tell you something even if it sounds like gibberish!
Olivia, Rothwell, mum to Eleni and Theo

I agree with trying not to worry too much about little things. Save the sharp 'NO' and raising your voice for real danger, then you know they might hear you in an emergency; don't let it be a background noise they hear all the time and tune out. Say 'Yes' a lot, with caveats such as: 'You can have x, as soon as you have done y', or for items they want, say, 'Yes, you can have that one day. Why don't you put it on your birthday/Xmas/wish list?'

The main thing for me with two littlies, and as an only child myself, has been to divide and conquer. Every day make sure you do something, even reading one page of a comic book, with each child separately, if at all possible. Send them off to separate rooms to get ready for school/ bed/going out, then they play up less and dawdle less, I get less stressed and have to yell, 'Hurry up' less, and sometimes they seem to enjoy each other's company more afterwards. I hope they will like each other when they grow up, at least some of the time. I am very conscious of being alone in the world myself.

Alison, North London, mum to Anna May, 6 and Hazel, 3

Listen to your children and respect their views and their concerns. Praise them for doing well and for good behaviour. Correct them when they are behaving badly. Fuel their imagination and find the child within yourself so that they think they have the most fun parent ever. Always find time – even if it is only ten minutes – to have a cuddle and talk about their day.

Toni, Walthamstow, mum to Chloe, 7 and Brandon, 2

Let them know clearly what you want; for instance, 'You need to sit down now' rather than 'Stop that!', or 'Put your hands on the table so I know you are listening' rather than 'Stop fiddling.' Sometimes children know what they shouldn't do, but not what they should. You can see it on *Supernanny*, etc. when the children are walking to school or demanding things inappropriately because they have never been told what is expected of them.

Praise, praise, praise, and don't sweat the small stuff! If a happy, joyful, positive atmosphere is the norm, then merely losing the smile can be enough to correct behaviour. If every day is miserable and full of negativity and admonishment, then it doesn't matter to them whether they behave or not.

Sarah, Hackney, mum to Aphra, 1 (and teacher of excluded secondary-school children)

Always tell them how much you love them. Build their confidence and self-esteem. A little 'how great you are' is a massive building-block in their self-esteem. Encourage-ment in all they do, knowing they have support from parents and siblings, brings out the best in them. For the older children, i.e. teenagers, still tell them how much you love them, but the biggie is communication. Always communicate – don't dictate! Be open and honest with them. I used to tell my kids, 'I may not always like what you tell me, but if it's the truth, then we can work on that and find a way to overcome hurdles in life.' I have two well-adjusted teenaged kids who will quite openly share anything with me. I didn't have that luxury as a teenager, so that's why I made a conscious decision to be totally open and honest with my children.

Ann, Co Tyrone, mum to Naomi, 20, Liam, 16 and Michael, 5

Why do siblings fight?

Does it seem that your children are always arguing, bickering or fighting over every little thing – which chair they sit on at the breakfast table, which way round the cornflakes box is facing . . . and so on until bedtime?

Eighty per cent of us have more than one child, so it's likely that we'll have to deal with some degree of sibling rivalry. There aren't many children who start out life as best friends, happy playing together for hours on end.

Older siblings tend to look at younger ones with irritation, while the younger ones look up to the older ones and want to imitate them and prove themselves to be equal to them. This is a recipe for disaster, especially when you add in the fact that as a parent you are the most important thing in their worlds, so they are both looking for your attention in whatever form that might take.

Each child is a unique individual, yet we often expect siblings to get on with each other and play regardless of personality type, gender, age and so on. This, in many ways, could be seen as unreasonable of us as parents but in reality it provides a golden opportunity for children to experiment and grow. Children need to learn about discord, about feeling uncomfortable, as this enables them to learn about negotiation, listening to their own and others' feelings and expressing points of view in the safety of the home environment, where, if necessary, their parents and other carers can help guide them through the trickier bits. Also, it is through these very first relationships that they learn about respecting themselves and each other and this is reinforced by the ways in which their parents help them to manage their burgeoning thoughts and feelings.

As grown-ups, it's our brothers and sisters who often provide us with the strongest bonds – our relationships with them can outlast all others and we often feel a special kinship. Even though your children are struggling now, it may all be worth it in the future!

If the rivalry is not too bad, don't worry. Some arguing and fighting is inevitable, and it's how they learn how to negotiate and learn about their place in the world. These tips (pp. 75–8) will help you, but be reassured that sibling rivalry is a normal part of family life.

If your children are constantly having a go at each other, it's probably affecting you too, and the family home will be a less happy place. Try to take the bull by the horns and see if you can start to calm things down. It won't be possible overnight, but you should see a change over a couple of weeks.

Ask the Netmums:
What do you do when your children fight?

I have three boys, aged five, three and one. Between tantrums, arguments and fighting, there's never a dull moment. How I deal with it depends on the issue. I try to delegate in some cases, ignore in others and sometimes let them sort it out for themselves. This behaviour is, after all, a normal part of growing up and learning how to get along (or not!). One or another may spend time on the bottom step or in their room, or the youngest gets put out of the room for a few seconds occasionally (he's seventeen months). If the issue is whose turn it is, then I tend to try to remember (sometimes unsuccessfully) whose turn it really is; if I can't remember, then I'll pick a reason why one of them is getting whatever rather than the other (who put their shoes away as asked, etc.). Sometimes if they can't share or take it in turns and the situation gets out of hand, then I just take away whatever is being fought over.

Shadow, Kettering, mum to Nayan, 5, Tallin, 3 and Ocean, 1

My youngest is the dominant one mainly because she gets physical. Ever since she learned that she could grab her sister's hair, that's what she's done whenever things aren't going her way. And she also has the attitude: 'it's not doing what I want – thump it!', which applies to toys, furniture and other people! When they bicker, she starts the hair pulling and the thumping. It takes a lot to make her older sister hit back now (she used to straight away), but she screams and yells and starts to threaten, 'I'm telling', which makes my younger daughter worse. Before you know it, they are fighting and rolling on the floor if you don't get to them in time. If we get to them in time, distracting them can help, but if it doesn't, we have to separate them for a while – never long, just long enough to calm them down. It's difficult because you never really know who started it or how. Of course, each will say it was the other one, and whom do you believe? Sometimes you can make a very good guess from knowing their past behaviour and what else is around them in the room (i.e. if elder daughter's Ello has gone flying across the room, you can bet your life that she was playing with it and the youngest came in, wasn't allowed to join in, and so sent it all flying), but because you are never 100 per cent sure, it's hard to know whether to punish one or both. Generally they end up in separate rooms until both calm down and we try to get them to apologise.

Sharron, Luton, mum to Louisa, 5 and Samantha, 2

I try to stay out of it unless they are really laying into each other, as I think it is important that they learn to sort things out themselves. Thankfully, it is very rare that they do fight because they really are the best of friends.

I do try to make them understand how the other person is feeling. For example, if Emma takes a toy from Sam, I'll ask Sam to take one off Emma and ask Emma how she feels, and this works well. It's not to show them tit for tat but to help them understand how others feel. They'll say sorry and swap back toys in no time!

We'll also distract them. If they are squabbling, we can tell it's because they are getting fed up, hot or tired, or whatever, so by introducing a new game or doing something silly it diffuses the situation before it escalates. I'll 'throw a tantrum' or lay down still in the middle of the floor and they'll forget any upset they were going to get into. Sam is also great at getting Emma to do what he wants now or, rather, getting her to do something other than what she wanted to do in the first place: he'll make another activity sound great to her so she does that instead. We can tell that our distraction methods have worked, as he is adopting them for himself!

Donna, Rotherham, mum to Samuel, 5 and Emma, 3

Ask yourself:

Could you make a little time to look and think?

You could start by taking a couple of days to watch what is happening. Jot down a few notes if you want, so you can review them properly afterwards. Try the ABC method as outlined above (see p. 53).

Antecedents: What started the fight? What was going on immediately before it happened? What are they fighting about?

Behaviour: What did the fight entail? Was there physical violence, snatching toys, etc.? What happens when they argue? Do they both start it, or is one child more demanding?

Consequences: Is it the child who is usually naughty that you automatically tell off first? Or is it the one who is loudest? Or are you reacting to the one who comes to you first? Do you treat your children differently? If one child (the youngest?) is getting more of your attention, the others will use all their imagination and every ounce of creativity to dream up new ways to get your attention.

When an argument or bickering starts, have a look at the big picture of what is going on: where you are sitting, who you are facing or talking to. What are you saying? What is your body language saying? Is the child who is behaving badly being rewarded for his behaviour by getting more of your attention?

Do problems happen at one time of day in particular? If there's one time of day that is difficult, can you diffuse the problems by feeding them a little earlier, getting them in the bath just before the trouble usually starts or heading it off by suggesting a run around the garden? If it's not that simple, read on!

Five peaceful practices

1. Sit down and have a chat with them

   Children as young as three can understand these discussions, but don't make them last forever! See if you can reach some agreements. Tell the children how their fighting makes *you* feel to start with, and that you want to work with them to see if you can make everyone happier.

   If your children's arguing sometimes results in violence, whether through frustration or malice, you might want to agree some family rules with them. Keep it simple: no kicking, no hitting, and perhaps no name-calling if they're good at trading insults.

   Agree you will need to take a 'zero tolerance approach' to breaking these rules, so it's two minutes on the bottom step whenever it happens. You might think that a ten year old is too big for 'bottom step' punishment, but it still works, even at that age! You'll need to be firm and calm and refer to the rules that they have talked about and agreed to.

2. When an argument starts

   You want them to start to sort out their own problems whenever possible, so next time they have an argument calmly listen to both sides. It takes time, but it's worth it. Don't be shocked by the intensity of the feelings that they are experiencing ('I hate her', 'I wish she was dead', 'I'm going to kill him' aren't unusual!) but try to get them to express themselves and, most importantly, show them that you understand and have noticed them.

   'Did you get cross when Joe didn't want to join in?'

'It sounds to me as though you're very frustrated. Do you feel like you've been waiting a long time for your turn?'

'Why did you scream? Was it because you are hurt or are you feeling mad at Susie?'

'You are both looking rather sad at the moment.'

'If you don't feel like talking at the moment, that's OK. We can wait a few minutes until you're ready.'

3. Help them to help themselves
    Having acknowledged their feelings and got them to say how they feel, it is time to see if you can help them generate their own solutions. If your children are highly competitive, perhaps you can encourage them to play more cooperative games?

    'Don't you think you will both feel better if you take it in turns? Do you want to borrow the kitchen timer to make sure it's completely fair?'

    'Because you make everything into a competition, there's always a winner and a loser, and that makes someone sad. Can we work together instead? Why don't we see if you can both work together to build the biggest tower possible within five minutes.'

    'If James is making too much noise in here for you to concentrate, do you think it might be a good idea for one of you to come and play next door instead?'

4. Build their confidence

As with all parenting, being positive with your children when they are being well behaved will reinforce the good behaviour. Help them to feel good about themselves. Look for ways to compliment them. 'Catch' them playing nicely together and say how lovely it is to see them having fun together – maybe you could ask to join in? Thank and praise them for starting to sort out their own arguments or for getting ready for school in the morning with no quarrelling.

5. Why it's worth persevering

You'll probably find things won't change overnight – they'll still be bickering and fighting a week on – but if you've taken the 'sting' out of it by then, you're doing well. Within a few weeks or a couple of months, hopefully it will be down to a reasonable level. The skills you teach them now will help them so much in later life. They will help them to control their anger when provoked, talk their way out of difficult situations and accept compromises. They will help them to understand others better and to be aware of their needs . . . and to be a good parent when their turn comes.

Recipe for successful parenting

If you want to succeed at parenting, aim to create a happy home rather than perfectly behaved children.

- Take a few parenting tips and techniques to suit your children's ages and stages.
- Add a great sense of humour.
- Sprinkle with a few crisis coping techniques.
- Combine that with a huge amount of patience.

- Fold in some acceptance that children are children and are naturally noisy and messy.
- Add a handful of understanding that challenging you is part of their learning to be independent little people.
- Mix all that up with loads and loads of love.

Be prepared to make mistakes and to forgive yourself when you get it wrong and to forgive your children when they get it wrong – and start all over again. Turn out a gorgeous, well-balanced, happy little person.

3 Tired and Emotional

Why, oh why, don't babies sleep? New mums (and mums of two, three and four year olds and more) are often so exhausted, we should hardly be in charge of a kettle, never mind a baby! Why is Mother Nature so unkind that in our fragile, post-labour stage she programmes our baby to ensure we don't get the sleep we need? And why does this continue for months and sometimes years? This is the $64 million question. And only Mother Nature knows the answer.

Wouldn't life be so much simpler and easier if babies slept? Wouldn't you have an extra baby or two if you knew you'd get eight hours' sleep each night? Imagine if babies and children had a little switch: On/Off. You could turn them on in the morning at about 8am, switch them off for an hour after lunch, then back on until bedtime at 8pm. And you could keep them turned off for an extra couple of hours on Sunday mornings.

If we could do that, kids wouldn't be such hard work at all. We'd be able to enjoy our children so much more because we wouldn't be so exhausted. We'd be able to spend quality time with our partners and have evenings out. Sure, we'd have occasional bad days, but we'd stay calm and not lose our grip, because we would have had our eight hours' sleep and the clock-off time would always be in sight. We'd cross the 8pm finish time and relax. We'd live well-planned and ordered lives.

Rrrinnnngg. Back to reality: babies that need to be jiggled and rocked from 7pm to 11pm every evening and then wake up every two hours for night feeds; evenings spent in front of Nick Jr. rather than *Coronation Street*; toddlers who refuse to go to bed; older children who keep coming downstairs because they can't sleep, or are scared of monsters; children who have nightmares; 6am starts and midnight finishes; tired, whingy children and exhausted grumpy parents.

This chapter focuses on some strategies for coping and some new ways of looking at the whole subject of babies and children and sleep.

Some Age-Related Issues

Little babies to six months

It could be helpful for you to think about and define the problem. Little babies do not naturally sleep long stretches at night at times that are convenient to us. Is it possible that the problem may be that your baby is sleeping well for her age and stage but her sleep routine doesn't suit your routine? We tend to think in terms of 'getting the baby to sleep', but is it possible that the baby is getting enough sleep but not in the hours that suit you? A good way to judge the situation is to decide if the child is getting enough rest and seems fairly happy all day.

For instance, if your baby is sleeping well from 8pm to 2am and then waking regularly for the rest of the night, and nothing seems to settle her, you may need to consider that she is getting her best sleep in those six hours and, just for now, you need to work to *her* schedule.

If you go to bed at 8pm and sleep well until 2am, you'll have had six solid hours of sleep, and if you manage to grab an extra couple of hours through the rest of the night you will be a lot less tired the next day. Going to bed at 8pm is boring and frustrating, especially when you've had a long day and are desperate for a little me-time. But there is truth in the old saying that an hour's sleep before midnight is worth two hours after.

Try not to feel resentful. Perhaps tape your favourite evening TV programmes and watch them when you're up early with the baby. Maybe take the baby into your bed and snuggle down together knowing that this is your special time. Most of all, remember that this phase doesn't last – it'll only be for a while and things will slowly readjust. The most important thing right now is that you get enough sleep to cope with life for you and your family.

It is also helpful to know that there are sleepy babies and wakeful babies. It's nothing you are doing or are not doing: some babies come into the world as little dormice, happy to snuggle down to sleep anywhere. There are also highly sensitive babies who need to feel cuddled all night and solid sleepers who will crash out anywhere and stay asleep all night. There are also owl babies and lark babies – just like grown-ups, some are at their best in the evening and some like early mornings (the old wives' tales say it depends on the time of day your baby is born). We all know someone who claims their baby goes down at 6pm and sleeps through until 8am, but it is unlikely to be anything wonderful they are doing. It's mostly luck. And you can console yourself with the thought that their second baby will be a screamer and what a shock they'll get then!

Every baby is different so try not to mould your baby to some generalised average. Work with your baby and try to read her signals. Every mum is different too. If you are happy to bring your baby into your bed and snuggle down to disturbed but cosy nights together, then go for it (read about safe co-sleeping on pp. 91–2). Don't let anyone tell you that what you are doing is wrong. If you can't cope with that and need to have a definite routine with baby in the cot, then that's fine too – some of the techniques below might help you. You need to find a balance between what is right for your baby and what is right for you.

Remember that your baby is very little and their current sleep pattern (or lack of one!) is a phase that will pass. It may be more trouble than it is worth to try to force your baby's pattern to suit yours. It might be worth adapting your routine, knowing that this is a relatively short phase.

Older babies

It is worth remembering that as adults when we fall asleep at night we rarely sleep right through to morning; we wake up several times but, because everything is the same as it was when we went to sleep, we turn over and go back to sleep and in the morning we don't even remember that we woke. You only have to think about what it is like for you when you sleep in a strange bed. During the night as you stir you wonder where you are and can become wide awake.

This holds true for babies too. Remember that whatever is associated with going to sleep may need to be repeated in order for them to be able to return to sleep. So, if you feed, rock or cuddle your baby to sleep and then put him in the cot, it is likely that you will need to do this again during the night when he or she stirs. Also, if the baby falls asleep in one place and is then transferred to the cot later, this again can be a cause of disturbed nights. So the key to night waking is often to be found in the settling routine.

It is helpful if you can help your baby to fall asleep in her cot without you being there. This will undoubtedly be easier for some babies than for others. You may need to take a step-by-step approach, but be responsive to what your baby needs.

1. Always try to put your baby in her cot awake. Obviously, very young babies often fall asleep with a feed. From the time that they are having three good meals a day, try separating the last milk drink from the bedtime settling. They should not be hungry in the night at this stage.
2. Stay with her until she falls asleep, at first stroking her face and singing to her.
3. Gradually reduce the time you spend doing this so that you leave the room when she is drowsy and knows that you are going. If she cries, go back to her and stroke her face so that she knows you are there but leave again when she is drowsy.
4. Eventually you will be able to put her in her cot and leave her to fall asleep alone.

If you are having problems, it might be useful to keep a diary of what happens each night so you can keep an eye on it. If you are worried in any way, or feel your child isn't settling for a reason other than lack of routine do contact your health visitor or GP for help and advice. If none of this helps and you are back at square one and at the end of your tether, read 'When all else fails' on p. 87.

Toddlers
Older babies and toddlers might not feel sleepy or be ready for sleep, but keep to a regular bedtime, otherwise you risk altering bedtime

every night depending on how tired your child is and then the routine goes out the window. You also risk your child becoming overtired and missing his sleep-slot.

> **When children miss their natural bedtime, to keep them awake their body releases extra hormones, such as adrenaline, which make them pumped up or 'wired' and make falling asleep difficult.**

It is well worth considering a few quiet activities your child can do in his bedroom on his own for a short while: a jigsaw, Lego, a story tape and so on. Obviously, this is only possible if circumstances and time permit, but it is a nice way of managing bedtime and of helping your child enjoy his bedroom and his own company at bedtime, so bedtime doesn't become a separation from you.

Timing

It is very important to get the timing of bedtime right. It's useless trying to get children to sleep when they are wide awake, but the clues that they are ready to go to sleep can be hard to spot. By the time they look sleepy and start yawning, it is often too late!

Some toddlers go into a calm and happy state, which indicates they are ready to fall asleep. Parents usually miss this, because who wants to put children to sleep when they are in such a lovely mood, cuddly and good company? Some can become really active and can be literally bouncing all over the place but will nevertheless drop off easily if put to bed while still bouncy. It can be worth paying close attention to the times when you do succeed in getting your child to sleep without too much work, and try to note what mood they were in just beforehand.

If you miss your chance and they get their second wind, you have to wait until they go into the next sleepy cycle and try again. A common mistake parents make is to notice that it is impossible to get their child to sleep at 7pm and take it to mean she needs a later bedtime, when actually maybe she needs an earlier bedtime and 7pm is too late. If you do miss the boat, you'll end up beating your head against the wall trying to get her to sleep, so it can be less stressful to let her get up, do a bit of reading or play some quiet games and try again later.

There is also a school of thought that says that the more children sleep, the more sleep they need. An expert called Marc Weissbluth, MD in a book entitled *Healthy Sleep Habits, Happy Child*, maintains that most parents tend to cut out naps when their child is too young, resulting in overtired children who can't settle down to sleep. Some parents feel their child needs less sleep than other children but it can be that these are the children who are actually sleep deprived, which is what results in their overactive behaviour. If you have cut out your child's nap, and then find he falls asleep in his buggy or the car, or can't quite make it till bedtime without getting really irritable then it is very possible that you have cut the nap out too soon.

Routine

It's always important to have a good bedtime routine even from the earliest days so that your baby learns that night and day are different. Human brains understand, remember and respond to patterns, so if you do the same thing each evening, i.e. a nice warm bath or wash, a feed, lights low and cuddles, a story, bed and soft low music or lullabies, it sends a strong signal to the brain that it's time to get ready for sleep. Baby massage is also an excellent way of helping babies and young children to relax and stay calm before sleep.

Many children, as they start to get older, feel afraid of the dark. Psychologists think that this might be because the mother switches off the light as she leaves the bedroom and darkness thus becomes associated with feelings of being abandoned. In order to prevent this from happening, you might think of switching the light off before it's time for you to leave the room. You could even potter about in the room tidying things away so that the dark becomes a friendlier place for your baby. Many sleep problems can be cured easily with some reassurance that nothing bad will happen to your child in the night. A nightlight or leaving the door open could make all the difference.

Rewarding positive behaviour

A star or reward chart for slightly older children can be a successful way of encouraging positive behaviour. Two stars can be earned each night: one star for going to bed nicely and then another for staying in bed until morning. See the section on star charts on p. 59 in Chapter 2, Children Behaving Badly.

The sleep fairy can be a useful ally. Tell your child that if she is very good at night, then in the morning the sleep fairy will have brought her a gift – something small that will be appreciated, such as a small car or a hair bobble. This reward system might be better linked to a star chart: the child gets a reward after earning however many stars. Dream up your own reward systems.

Substitutes

A special teddy, a 'guardian angel', a little fairy statue . . . try to introduce one of these to your child as a symbol of being looked after while he sleeps. A little plug-in nightlight might be the glow of the sleep fairy's wings. Or maybe use a little torch that the child can keep under the pillow and 'control'.

When all else fails

Babies cry because it is their one way to get our attention and to communicate with us. To start off with, ask yourself, 'Why is my baby crying?' Check that he's not too hot or too cold, that he is clean and dry, and that he is comfortable. Sometimes when we've been through the usual checklist, we don't know why the baby is crying and this can make us feel helpless in the face of a young baby's distress.

It is generally accepted that from six months of age, babies are quite capable of sleeping through the night, but, as we know, ours doesn't! And there is so much conflicting advice that our poor tired brains hit overload and we end up crying with exhaustion and frustration.

The two techniques that can be used for solving sleep problems are:

1. Controlled crying
2. Gradual retreat

Controlled crying

Since recently published new research on baby brain development, there has been a lot of controversy over controlled crying. During the first year of life, nerve endings in the baby brain are making zillions of new connections and develop at an astounding rate. The brain more than doubles in weight during this time. Good interaction with the baby affects the growth positively and stress has a negative impact.

The scientific research into the effects of controlled crying are largely contradictory. Recently, the Australian Association for Infant Mental Health suggested that controlled crying should not be used until the child is three years old, whereas other studies show there is no evidence that it harms the child in any way.

Controlled crying is a planned intervention. It is about helping your child to settle to sleep on her own. This entails leaving her after settling her down in her usual routine. If she cries, then return to her after two minutes at first, then four minutes, then five. When the parent returns each time, they gently and silently lay the child down, tuck her in and stroke or pat her for a short time and then walk away again.

How easy it sounds! How difficult it is to put into practice is almost impossible to describe. Your child will likely cry and scream and beg you to lift him and hold him and cuddle him. If he does, then give him a cuddle but do not remove him from the cot. Do not turn your back on a very distressed child. There may be other reasons why he is so very distressed. Try to figure out what is going on for him. Have there been upheavals in family life, such as a new baby? Are you and your partner happy? Is there a new partner? Has he started nursery?

You need to be very sure that there is no other way you can deal with the problem other than using controlled crying and you need to be really determined before you start.

Those that are most successful with this technique are those who, quite frankly, are at the end of their tether and cannot go on as they are. If you are at that stage, then choosing this technique does not make you a bad parent – it actually might make you a better one. If you know that you can't carry on as you are, then you are at the stage where you simply won't be able to give your child the best care and attention in other areas of his life. In fact, you may start to resent your child or you may end up physically or mentally ill. If you can crack the sleep problem, your child will get the best out of his parents – and that's a good thing. Desperate times deserve desperate measures. So if you are feeling desperate, this could be the method for you.

You need to be determined and make sure your partner or another adult is with you to support you. Some parents have done this successfully using a sleep diary and recording what they have done along the way. Often they have made the leaving-to-cry time much shorter, depending on their tolerance levels. The only stipulation is that it has to get longer each time. Most mums who have started – and followed through – the programme agree that it usually takes three nights (three very hard nights) to crack it.

Gradual retreat

Another solution that is gentler, but requires endless patience over at least a two-week period, is the gradual retreat method. This involves putting your child to bed and sitting by the cot or bed. You must become the most boring mum you can possibly be. If she speaks or tries to engage you, keep repeating the same phrase – something like, 'Sssshhh, shhhhh, settle down. No more talking now.' Do this for two nights. On the third night, move a few feet away and do exactly the same thing. Every two nights move further away. You'll end up by the door, outside the door, at the top of the stairs, halfway down the stairs, in the hallway, in the lounge, etc. If your child resists one night, move back to the previous position until they are comfortable with it and then carry on. Do the same thing if the child wakes in the night (yes, that's the very hard bit). And don't give up halfway through – you will usually have a result within two weeks. Before you start, accept that for the next two weeks, there is no point scheduling any evening TV or other activities – it'll only be more frustrating for you if you are hoping to have them asleep by a certain time.

Babies in the bed?

This is a topic designed to produce a great old argument! As with all things related to parenting, at the end of the day it is about looking at the facts, then making a decision that suits you.

In many countries, it is normal for families to share beds and for babies and toddlers to co-sleep with their mothers. In fact, there are lots of 'underground' co-sleeper mums in this country who don't admit to sleeping with their babies for fear of being criticised. We say, 'Go for it! Come out of the closet. Stand up and be counted.' The image of mum and dad in bed, the baby asleep in her cot and the toddler happily asleep in his own room is like the image of the family with 2.4 kids and a picket fence. How common is it really?

Do what works for you and yours. There are homes where dad sleeps in the spare room, or where they have abandoned the bed and instead have two king-sized mattresses on the floor. There are homes where everyone goes to bed at 8pm, or where no one goes to bed until 11pm. Go with the flow, do what works for you, and remember that each phase is a passing phase.

If family members (grandmothers, usually!) criticise you for bringing your baby into your bed, you can tell them that for millions of years mums have slept with their babies, and in many cultures it is still the norm. In fact, it is only in recent years and only in 'civilised' western society that we began to create separate sleeping rooms and spaces for our children. Indeed, the SIDS (Sudden Infant Death Syndrome) Global Task Force showed recently that low SIDS rates are associated with the highest co-sleeping rates.

And there is evidence that mothers of breastfeeding babies who sleep with their babies will be less tired, as their sleep cycle synchronises with their baby so that the mum is woken only when both are in the light stages of sleep rather than being dragged from deep REM sleep.

There are, of course, guidelines to protect the child and, once you've checked those out, you should both sleep happily together. Enjoy snuggling up with your warm little bundle.

Essential safety advice

1. Don't sleep with your baby if you have been drinking or taking drugs or medication that makes you drowsy.
2. Don't let the pillows get near the baby.
3. Don't let the baby sleep between two adults.
4. Use sheets and blankets instead of a quilt so that the baby doesn't risk overheating.
5. Make sure that there is no gap between the mattress and the wall where the baby could get caught.

6. Don't sleep on a sofa or chair with your baby as he may get squashed into a corner.
7. If you have the baby on the open side of the bed, either use a suitable bed-guard or have a mattress or pillows on the floor in case the baby falls out.
8. Always put your baby on his back to sleep as you would in a cot.

An alternative might be something like the BedNest crib, which is an innovation that allows a baby to sleep beside Mum but not quite in the same bed (see www.baby-crib.co.uk). It allows mother and baby to be within breathing and touching distance and provides a great alternative to bed sharing for anyone who, for whatever reason, finds bed sharing unsuitable.

There is conflicting advice about sharing a bed with a baby under twelve weeks old. If you have any concerns, discuss them with your GP or health visitor.

Other possible reasons your baby isn't sleeping

Night terrors/nightmares

With nightmares, the dream takes place during lighter sleep, usually during the second half of the night. The child wakes up crying and calling out. If children are frightened by a dream, then they need reassurance to be able to calm down and go back to sleep. The best thing is to do this with the minimum of disturbance to yourself and the child. Don't leave them too long in the hope that they will go back to sleep. Sit on the bed or get in with them and cuddle up, stroke their hair and make soothing noises. Tell them they are safe. The child will be aware of you and find your presence reassuring.

Sometimes a nightmare is a reaction to a change in routine or any change at all. It is the mind trying to work it all out and get to grips with it. Younger children may not have the language to be able to tell you what happened and will not understand the concept of a dream. To them it was reality, which is why it is so hard for them to go back to sleep. Your child will need you to hold her tightly and reassure her.

Night terrors are different to nightmares. They occur in the deepest part of a child's sleep. Sometimes a child can seem awake, with eyes wide open but still be dreaming and calling out. They can be difficult to wake and seem very distressed. It can be a little scary for you to see your child like this, especially as they seem to be very frightened but appear to be unaware of their surroundings and unresponsive to your attempts to comfort and reassure. Stay calm and quiet, as shouting to try to wake them can increase their fear. It can also be unhelpful to say 'there is nothing there' as the terror seems very real to them. Instead of trying to wake them up, try 'getting into their dream'. For example, if they are afraid of something (a monster or bee or spider?) try opening the window and chasing it out. Close the window behind it and say loudly, 'There. It's gone.' Once calmed, they will return to sleep quite quickly and are no longer frightened when fully awake. Seeing monsters is quite common and children need to know how to deal with them.

If your baby or toddler isn't sleeping, maybe keep a little sleep diary for a week. Jot down your routine and your little one's behaviour and show it to your GP or health visitor. There are sometimes medical causes for sleep problems (it is relatively rare but it is posssible) and the background information will be of great value.

Colic

Colic is when a healthy, well fed baby cries for more than three hours per day, more than three or four days per week without any obvious cause. It used to be thought of as a stomach or digestive disorder but while wind may contribute it isn't thought to be the cause of the crying. Sadly, as with the common cold, experts have yet to agree the cause, but they all agree they haven't found a cure. Many experts believe it is due to the baby having a particularly sensitive temperament, which may well be why evenings are worse, as the baby has absorbed so many stimuli throughout the day he's unable to calm down.

Before you decide your baby has colic, see your GP or health visitor and check that it isn't something else, such as silent reflux, which occurs when acidic juices back up (or reflux) from the stomach into the baby's oesophagus and digestive tract. The baby then swallows the acid back down, causing pain twice.

Although colic isn't a serious medical condition, hearing your doctor or health visitor dismiss it as 'just' colic can be bewildering. It underestimates just how stressful a baby with colic can be for new parents. Watching and hearing this tiny baby that you love so much crying in pain and being unable to help causes huge distress. And we are programmed to respond to a baby's cry. After three hours of listening to a baby scream our nerve endings are jangling and most mums are close to screaming themselves.

No advice on sleeping will seem helpful if you have a baby with colic. Indeed, a book with a paragraph or two on the condition but no solutions will make you want to hurl the book against the wall. Go on, it might help a tiny bit!

Colic is usually at its worst in the evening. Indeed, mothers in the sixties referred to the time between about 6pm and 8pm as 'the crying time'. If at all possible, have someone with you in the evenings – just for these few difficult weeks – and take it in turns to be with the baby. One goes upstairs and walks around with the baby while the other watches TV very loudly downstairs! By doing 'shifts' you will both stay calmer and better able to cope.

If your partner is at work, you don't have a partner or you have no friends or family around, and your baby is crying incessantly, you need to give yourself little breaks. Say, every fifteen minutes, put the baby down in a safe place, probably in the cot, and go into another room or the garden (ideally somewhere you can't hear the screams) and take some deep breaths. Have a cup of tea or a hot chocolate. Although it is tempting when you are so stressed to have a glass of wine, it is probably better not to. Alchohol is a depressant and might make you feel worse. Maybe wait until the baby has settled to sleep or another adult is home.

Remember that you won't be doing your baby any harm by leaving him for a few minutes – you will do more good, as when you pick him up again you'll be calmer and he'll feel that calmness.

If you feel really stressed and can't stand the noise any longer, call someone. Just hearing the sound of an adult voice can be helpful. If you can't think of anyone to call, call the Cry-sis helpline. This is a charity run by parents who have been at the end of their tether with crying babies and who now provide a service where you can talk to someone to help you through the worst moments. Call 08451 228 669; they're available from 9am to 10pm seven days a week. It's not a sign of weakness or failure to call them: they know that the sound of a screaming baby can, quite literally, drive you mad. Or log on to the Netmums Coffeehouse, where there is always someone to talk to online for a bit of support or advice.

The best advice is:

- Medical experts suggest that breastfeeding mothers stop drinking cow's milk as the baby may be having trouble with the protein in the cow's milk going through the breast milk.
- Movement: rocking, walking up and down, pushing the baby in the pram, or driving around in the car.
- Join a baby massage class. You will learn ways of interacting with your baby that will help you both feel more relaxed.
- Sucking can be helpful. Keep a breastfed baby on the breast all evening if necessary, or try a dummy if you haven't already.
- Tell yourself every day that this will not last. It rarely lasts beyond three months. Also remember that you are doing your absolute best – no mother could do more for your baby – and colic does not cause any lasting emotional or physical damage.
- Lots of mums report that cranial osteopathy has been very helpful. This is a very gentle manipulation of the bones of the skull which may have been 'squished' (for want of a better word) during childbirth and may be worth considering if your baby had a difficult entry into the world.
- To help relieve colic, try a positive touch routine (see below) a couple of times a day.

Positive touch

Be sure to relax before you start. The parents' relaxation technique goes like this:

- Sit comfortably.
- Take three deep breaths in and out; become aware of any body tension.

- Roll the shoulders back several times and then forwards to release them.
- Drop the head towards the chest and roll it from side to side to release the neck.
- Clasp the hands together, straighten the arms and push the palms of the hands out in front of you and then stretch the arms up to the ceiling, hold for a few seconds and then release.
- Make a fist with the hands, then open the hands and stretch the fingers wide several times to release and relax the hands.

Now you are ready to begin.[1]

- Lie the baby on his back on a towel lightly rolled around his body to encourage feelings of safety and security.
- The baby may be clothed or unclothed, but if unclothed expose only the area to be stroked.
- Use baby oil to stroke gently around the baby's abdomen in a clockwise direction about five times.
- Pause and bring the baby's knees up towards the abdomen and hold for a few seconds.
- Repeat for as long as the baby is happy for it to happen.

Possibly incorporate touch relaxation on legs into the routine: pull your baby's leg through your palms and fingers, hand over hand, from the thigh to foot.

Ask the Netmums:

How did you get your baby or children into a good sleep routine?

(1) These techniques are adapted from V. McClure, *Infant Massage: A Handbook for Loving Parents*, 3rd ed. (Bantam Books, New York, 2000)

If it feels like something 'isn't working', make sure you have a realistic expectation of what is achievable for you and your children and that it is based on sound knowledge. Try to remember that as your baby grows, she will be constantly changing. What happened last week might give little indication of what you are experiencing in the present. You'll find all too soon things drop into place and you'll wonder why you were so worried.

Focus on the positive things. For example, my little one has taken to solids like a duck to water: he's gone from fully breastfeeding to three meals a day in four weeks and loved everything I have given him. On the negative side, I could get focused on him waking in the night, but because I don't expect him to sleep through when he is so little it isn't a big problem. I also know that the 'medical definition' of 'through the night' is five hours, which most nights he manages from about 11pm to 4am, and that 'sleeping through' is technically impossible as we all wake periodically and dropping back to sleep again is something that needs to be learned. Finally, I also know that little ones have their startle reflex during sleep to prevent them from sleeping too deeply for too long, which is linked to the work that's been done on SIDS.
Claire, Northampton, mum to Harry, 8 months

I used controlled crying with all three children, but not until I was on my knees with exhaustion and my health visitor had tattooed on my forehead, 'An eleven-month-old baby does not need to breastfeed all night!' I have to say it worked like a charm. I was too soppy to do the more extreme version. I couldn't leave them crying for five or ten minutes and do nothing, so I invented my own version, which meant I went in frequently and just stroked them but

didn't pick them up. What they say about the five-day rule is absolutely true. The first day is bad, the second and third are a big improvement, the fourth is total hell and the fifth day you wake up in a panic because they've slept through! I was really loath to do it the first time round. To be honest, I thought it the height of cruelty, but fortunately I had an attentive health visitor who could see what a mess I was in. I trusted her judgement implicitly in every other area, so I reluctantly decided to have a go. The one thing I would say is that once you start you have to go through with it. Changing the rules will confuse your baby and you could end up with an even more wakeful baby.
Christine, Kingston, mum to Isabelle, 8, Aimee, 6 and Ethan, 3

I used well-known childcare expert Gina Ford's routines and my daughter became an angel overnight. She went from colicky screaming and short one- to two-hour naps to being happy and gurgly and sleeping for a full four to five hours at night at just two weeks old. At nine weeks, she was sleeping through. Everyone kept telling me to let her set the routine, but she was so unhappy – as was I – that I bit the bullet and tried a strict routine with her and it was bliss!
Tracy, Wolverhampton, mum to Maia, 2 and Cadence, 2 weeks

When our son was small, there were nights when I honestly thought I would never get to go to sleep again. I would be sitting there at two o'clock in the morning with a 'playful' baby, thinking, 'What on earth have I done wrong?!'

When he was first born, he slept in a Moses basket, but if he woke up I'd bring him into our bed and breastfeed him.

At first this was fine, as once he was asleep I would just put him back into his Moses basket. But as he got bigger and heavier, it got more and more difficult to move him into his Moses basket without waking him. We actually had one night where he did not go to sleep at all – we were walking the streets with him at midnight trying to get him to go to sleep. The baby finally went to sleep at about 6am, but my husband was late for work because he didn't wake when his alarm clock went off! Anyway, our son made his own sleep routine in the end – at about nine months he started sleeping through the night by himself most nights, but I can't actually pinpoint that it was anything we did that helped him do this.

I think the biggest mistake we made with his sleeping was bringing him into our bed, as he started to wake just so he could spend the rest of the night there. I also think the best thing we did with his sleeping routine is we brought his (very late) bedtime forward to 8 o'clock and increased the naps he had in the daytime. This seemed to help him get to sleep a lot more easily, and maybe contributed to him sleeping through the night.

Fran, Southeast London, mum to Benjamin, 1

Aki was breastfed since coming home from the hospital. He would always fall asleep on the boob, and then I would let him lie on my chest or put him down on the sofa during the day and in his cot at night. I kept this up until he was about seven months old. Once solids were firmly established, I wanted to stop the night feeds, as I had read that the baby wouldn't need them any more. I talked it over with my health visitor and she confirmed that Aki was most likely waking only because of habit. To break the habit, I decided to go with controlled crying, as I didn't see how else he would stop. This was quite hard work and took about three to four weeks before it was working properly.

I didn't have the heart to go about it by the book and increase the times by five minutes at a time, so I opted for shorter times increased only by a minute at a time. This is probably why it took longer to work, but I kept my sanity in the process. Aki got used to not being fed when he first woke around midnight fairly easily. The real struggle was dealing with the waking in the early morning, around 4am, when I would be yanked out of deep sleep and he would feel hungrier and not settle very easily. Surprisingly, Aki's father found this harder to deal with; I guess because he felt less in control than I did. He just had to listen to his son cry without really being able to help (even though I wasn't feeding Aki at night any more, he wouldn't be settled by anyone else). I made it a rule (more for myself than anything) that Aki wasn't allowed a feed until 6am, and he eventually got used to this and started waking at 6 on the dot. Then I would pick him up and put him in our bed, and we would both fall asleep while feeding. I kept up these morning feeds in bed until Aki was 15 months old, when it became more hassle than it was worth.

Aged 18 months, Aki still wakes up at about 6–6.30am each morning, but now drinks his milk out of his cup in the cot and still usually falls asleep for a bit longer. When he wakes up properly, at about 8–8.30am, he plays in the cot on his own for up to an hour while Mummy and Daddy sleep a bit longer. On weekends we sometimes still put Aki in our bed, but he tends to climb down to play with his toys on the bedroom floor.

Looking back, I'm fairly happy with the way we have gone about Aki's sleeping: he goes to sleep on his own in the evening after a story and a bit of milk and usually sleeps through. If he does wake up in the middle of the night, he usually settles again after a quick pat on the back and a kiss on the head. The controlled crying has left us untraumatised, and I would use it again on my future children if they showed no sign of letting go of night waking on their own.

Jutta, North London, mum to Aki, 18 months

I wish I'd known about co-sleeping when Sam was born, as it would have saved so many sleepless nights. I was lucky when Sam was first born that my husband worked part time and so had days free to cope if I'd been up all night and needed to catch up on my sleep the next day. Alex would also take Sam out of our room at night and sit with him curled up asleep on his chest for hours while listening to music and playing the computer in another room – this is a lovely memory for Alex now, all those quiet nights just him and his boy!

When things finally got too much and Sam would not settle by himself, we tried loads of different methods: staying in his room but not giving him attention, tucking him back in and firmly saying, 'No', moving out of the room one metre at a time and so on. Finally we came to controlled crying and that was a nightmare. I honestly didn't believe Sam would ever stop crying with us going into his room every five minutes, ten minutes, etc. It was never-ending and heartbreaking for us all. So – and I do feel cruel about this now – we put him to bed one night and left him to cry. He cried for forty-five minutes solid and then stopped dead and slept through; the next night he cried for fifteen minutes and the third night not at all. As I said, though, I wish I'd known it was fine, even normal, to share a bed – I would have done that – but hindsight is a wonderful thing!

Emma was a very good baby to start with and would wake for a breastfeed and go straight back into her cot no problem until she was about seven months old, when she became a nightmare, waking every twenty minutes for a breastfeed and I was at my wits' end and completely exhausted. I remember coming home from an evening Christmas shopping with my mum, walking into the kitchen and collapsing in tears because I didn't want to come home. I couldn't see the point if I was going to spend all night breastfeeding and not get any sleep. That night Alex took charge and he and I slept downstairs on the settee so that he could go and settle her without me being around with my milk. We prepared ourselves for even less sleep for a few days until she got used to the new routine. We thought it would be hell and even warned the neighbours. We still don't believe it, but she slept through that first night – no murmur, no night-time feed, nothing. She must have been waking up because we were there and maybe waking her up as we moved in bed. We ended up sleeping on the front-room floor for two weeks while we redecorated the attic bedroom for Sam and Sam's room for Emma. And she still is a little madam!

Donna, Rotherham, mum to Samuel, 5 and Emma, 3

We never tried to be quiet when they slept from day one, so they got used to everyday noises around them. If they woke during the night while still in a cot, we would lie them down and gradually withdraw from their room, but we didn't get

them out. As toddlers, if they came into our room, we would return them to their own bed and tell them they could come back when it was morning. If it was light, we used to let them get in with us. They are both good sleepers now. This could be just how they are, or may be due to some of the above?
Lindsay, Sidcup, mum to Ella, 10 and Libby, 4

I was so lucky with the older two, as they slept right through really early on. My little one is a bit harder, bless him. I have almost got it sussed now that he wakes only for a drink, so instead of getting him up and giving him cuddles and milk, he is offered water or juice and is not picked up. I hold his bottle for him. He takes a couple of sips and goes back down now he knows he won't get milk. I have always made a point of hoovering and things when they are sleeping so they get used to the noise.
Jacqui, Peterborough, mum to Liam, 7, Zack, 5 and Ellis, 10 months

With my three, I have used the same routine. It was a case (when small) of a bath, getting changed in their own room and, immediately after getting them ready, putting a classical CD on very quietly and breastfeeding them in their room with no/little conversation, just hugs. Once they had finished their feed, I then laid them quietly in bed and left. Luckily, they haven't been bad at sleeping. If they wake, I tend to them but do not lift them out of bed; I calm them down by placing my hand on them gently, wait till they have calmed and leave. I have never had them in bed with me. We have always had a really good routine. Thankfully, we have no tears at bedtime and they accept that it is bedtime.
Deborah, Halifax, mum to Kelsey, 8, Luke, 5, and Cameron, 2

Getting into a routine early on helps – as does expecting to be woken up! We bathed, then massaged, then fed, then put to bed from early on – always carrying out the evening routine in the nursery in dimmed light and quiet. We used lavender oil in massage oil; it has to be very dilute for babies, so get specially blended oil if you are not sure about aromatherapy.

Be relaxed yourself, and don't stress when the routine changes, as it invariably does just when you think you have cracked it! And be aware that when people say that their babies 'sleep through' this may mean they sleep from midnight to 5am not from 7pm to 7am! It does get easier as the child gets older. Sticking to a routine has worked for us. Max, now nearly two, sleeps in his proper bed from 7pm to 7am and does not get up unless he is ill. Toby is settling into his routine and we hope will prove to be as good a sleeper as big bro'!

Emma, South Elmsall, mum to Max, 22 months and Toby, 3 months

After twelve miserable weeks with my daughter, I gave up trying to get her to sleep in her cot. We moved a single bed next to the double. My daughter and I shared the double till she was about eighteen months, with my husband on my other side in the single. Then we switched to my daughter on the single, us on the double. When she was three and a half, we decorated her room and moved her and her bed and bedding into it – easy! We co-slept with my son from day one and saved ourselves the twelve weeks of aggro.

Katherine, London, mum to Rachel and Tom

4 Mums and Lovers

The children come first. As long as the children are happy, that's all that matters. Right? Well, actually, there is good evidence that if we want to do the best for our children, we should be putting our relationship with our partner first. It has been shown that in families where parents take care of themselves and their relationship, children fare better than children whose parents are neglecting both themselves and each other. This has real implications for our homes and family: it seems that going out for dinner with your husband – or finding other ways to have a bit of quality time together – can be contributing to your children's happiness and long-term success. So, if you need one, that's a pretty big motivator for wanting to make your relationship with your partner a little better.

It's too easy to muddle along together, assuming that once in love, always in love. And if things aren't great, well, we're so busy right now and we're too tired to do anything but slump on the sofa in the evenings anyway. Next year, we think, when the baby is a bit older, when things have settled down a little, then we'll spend some time on each other. But, of course, next year brings its own set of new challenges and reasons to be exhausted. In many ways, we seem to pass each other like ships in the night. We grunt instructions at each other, bump into each other in the bathroom occasionally and pass each other in the hall on the way in or out. The problem is that when we do eventually get a chance to spend time together, we may find we've lost that closeness we once had. One day the children will be gone, and we'll look up and it'll be only the two of us at home – and we might find we don't even know each other any more.

Of course, it's true that when our children are very young we have much less time and energy for each other. And when we are exhausted from broken nights and never-ending demands from toddlers, running a home and holding down a job, if someone suggests that what our relationship needs is candle-lit dinners and black negligees, we're likely to throw the book at their head!

The five relationship wreckers

Watch out for these relationship wreckers. They creep into your home and wreak havoc with your relationship and you don't even realise they are there . . . Stamp them out!

1. Resentment

Resentment is a horrible little worm (along the lines of a tapeworm), which finds mums with young children a wonderfully accepting host creature. This worm creeps in as a tiny baby worm, unseen by the naked eye. Often it creeps in when we are pregnant, before our baby is even born. *We* are the ones who feel sick and tired, *we're* the ones who get big fat tummies and swollen ankles, and *we* are the ones who can't continue to go to the pub with our friends at the weekend. His life doesn't seem to change; he can carry on as normal, not even seeming to think that what we are going through is a big deal. That's it – the worm is in.

And very slowly, it grows. And it grows. It feeds on anything in its path. It doesn't need huge sustaining meals (like an affair), it's perfectly happy to snack continually on little things: an overflowing bin not taken out; a week's worth of his clothes suddenly shoved into the laundry basket; another disturbed night with the baby or toddler while he snores beside you; (another) night out in the pub with his friends; money spent on football tickets; the fact that he has to be asked to take *his* children to the park or swimming on a Saturday. The resentment worm also thrives on throw-away comments: 'That dinner wasn't one of my favourites', 'The house is such a mess', 'There's nothing to eat.'

Resentment is a bit like that other destructive emotion, jealousy. It starts to cloud your vision and judgement – you start to read too much into things, take hurt where it isn't intended – and it can, over a period of time, destroy love.

Ask yourself:

What do you feel resentful about?

Imagine every time you give head space to those resentful feelings you are providing a fine meal for the resentment-worm, allowing it to grow stronger. And every time you choose not to feel resentful but to do something positive about it instead you are starving the worm and it will eventually die. Choose to think of something positive: a time you were really happy together, a time you had fun together, a time he supported you when you needed him. You can choose your feelings.

2. Blame

Does your home have a blame culture? Is something always someone's *fault*? Are you content only when you've attributed blame to someone? Blame should be apportioned only when someone has wilfully, knowingly and intentionally done something to upset or hurt someone else.

Next time your partner is to blame for something, ask yourself: did he do it intentionally and wilfully? Did he mean to hurt and upset me? Does it really matter that much? Is it something I can let go of? If it is something that needs to be addressed, such as a safety issue, then, of course, you must do so. But can you address it from a desire to achieve a good outcome (such as an agreement to how this situation will be handled in future) rather than wanting to prove him wrong and make sure he takes the blame?

3. Mummy-martyrdom

It's so easy to fall into this trap. You talked with your partner about joint parenting, about new men and modern-day fathers and how each person would have his or her role and each would be as important as the other and then, somewhere along the line, you forgot that and you took over. Maybe you felt in those very early days that it was 'my' baby. Or maybe you slipped into the powerful pattern set by your mum that the women in your family always looked after home and family while the men did men-things. Or maybe you didn't know how to ask for help. For whatever reason, you've ended up with a case of mummy-martyrdom. Instead of saying how you feel about it not being fair that you do all the night feeds, you sigh deeply, and get up full of resentment. The next day you sigh again, look miserable and say how tired you are. If your partner offers to help, you say in a clipped voice, 'No, thanks', while looking as if this may well be your last day on earth. You constantly say things like: '*I'll* do it', 'It's easier if *I* do it' and, all men's pet hate when they ask what's wrong, 'I'm fine', when you're plainly not!

Say what you mean. Don't expect him to guess or to interpret your sighs. He either won't notice, or will choose not to notice. It doesn't mean he doesn't care but, unless you explain, he won't understand. Try to be clear and as unemotional as possible, so instead of 'I'm completely exhausted. I don't think I can do this any more', try simply asking: 'I could really do with a night's sleep. Will you do the night shift tonight and I'll do tomorrow?' Instead of sighing and moping, sit down for a coffee and say, 'I've been a bit miserable recently because [tell him why]. Will you . . . [What would help you? A hug? A day out with your friends?]' Try to be specific about what would help and don't say, 'More help from you.'

Instead of saying, 'I'm fine', use the true meaning of the word, which is:

Fed up
Insecure
Neurotic
Emotional

Ask yourself:

How do you contribute to your partner not helping you?

For example: by not asking for what you need, criticising his help (he dressed the children but nothing matches, he made tea but it isn't healthy, he washed up but didn't finish the job). What can I ask my partner for that would help me most? How can I phrase it positively? ('Will you . . . ?')

4. Point scoring
Do you have a balance sheet in your relationship that isn't of the

financial kind? The one that goes like this . . . He stayed out late, three points for me. He had a lie-in, two points for me. I (sigh) got the car tax because he was never going to get round to it, two points for me. We had sex, three points for me . . . and so on. It's an unspoken and invisible balance sheet but it's always there. It hangs in the very air between you. And you always make sure you are heavily in profit while he is running at a continual loss. As you can see, it's a very close cousin of mummy-martyrdom: if you are prone to one, you are probably also afflicted with the other. If you must have a balance sheet, aim to make it balance! Imagine that in a successful relationship you will each have earned and used up the same number of points. He gets a lie-in on a Saturday – two points; you go to the hairdresser on a Saturday afternoon – two points. You get the car tax – two points; he reads the bedtime stories – two points. Stop feeling superior. Get back on equal terms. Use up your points and enjoy them!

5. 'Why should I?'

All but very mild-mannered mums will be asking at this point: 'Why should I make all the effort? We're both grown-ups. Why should I have to treat him like a child and use what in many ways are parenting techniques on him? Why should men get away with being treated like children?' There are three answers to that:

a) We are all human. Women, children and, yes, dads too, need the same things in life. After food, water and air, we need:
   – to be loved, not ridiculed, criticised or put down;
   – to be needed, not overlooked and put aside;
   – to be successful, not feel like a failure.
b) We can't change other people, but we can change ourselves and our reactions to other people. Often by doing that, we change the atmosphere and, in turn, their behaviour changes too. By changing our approach, we may see positive changes in our

partners and our relationship and in the general mood and atmosphere of our homes.

c) By making an effort in your relationship, you will also benefit. Your relationship is not a battleground where only one of you can win. The aim here is that you both win.

Ask the Netmums:

What drives you mad about your other half?

He's always right and he has never cleaned the bathroom in six years of togetherness. He says he has, but why don't men understand that a quick squirt of the Toilet Duck is not cleaning the bathroom!? Another thing . . . why don't men understand that when you are crying what you need is to be held, not for someone to ask (incredulously), 'What's up now?' He has lots of good points, however. Lucky for him, or I would've been off years ago!
Juliet, Scarborough, mum to James, 15 months

The biggest things he does that annoy me are having to ask him to do anything, and he'll carry on watching telly, and taking half an hour to bath the kids – that's half an hour to psyche himself up to do it, not actually do it! It would be quicker for me to do it myself, but it's the principle! And he thinks spending quality time with the kids is when they're in the same room as him while he's watching TV!
Tina, Kent, mum to Saffron, 20, Simon, 18, Daisy, 2½, and full-time stepchildren, Jessica, 10, and Fleur, 9

He still has a little bit of our pre-children life and I don't. He goes out to work and gets to socialise and see friends. I

would never stop him going and actually encourage it, but it's the one thing that I don't like. I guess I am just jealous!
Claire, Cheshire, mum to Max and Thomas, 3

Clothes on the floor, stubble around the sink, snoring, never remembering anything I've said . . . I could go on all night!
Joanna, Bristol, mum to Alannah, 10, and Johnny, 7

Living with him is sometimes like living with someone under water! I seem to be talking to a brick wall most of the time. He is really great with my daughter and is hard working, but it's the usual 'don't make time for each other' thing!
Fiona, Aberdeen, mum to Annabel, 2

He never gets up with my little one when he is on a day off. I would love to get a lie-in but because he gets up early for work every other day he needs his lie-in! The fact that I get up with Sam every day is irrelevant!
Michelle, Bournemouth, mum to Samuel, 1

He never tidies up after himself, leaves underwear on the bedroom floor, never changes the loo roll, goes on the computer far too much, he is sooooo unromantic . . . better stop or else I may start to wonder why the hell I am with him! Love him really!
Claire, Norwich, mum to Jayden, 16 months

I know I agreed to be the housewife. I know he is the 'breadwinner', but I feel he could at least try to do some bits around the house. He works incredibly hard and then moans at me when the house is a mess and I've still not finished unpacking since our last house move, but he

doesn't seem to realise just how hard I work too! Leaving empty milk cartons on the worktop . . . what's that about? Why can't he put them in the bin? Putting the sugar cup back in the cupboard when it's empty! Is it really so hard to refill it?! I guess it's silly things, and feeling I'm not appreciated as I feel I should be. I love him really, though!
Teresa, Heywood, Rochdale, mum to Sammie-Jo, 4, Charlie, 3 and George, 19 months

He's always hungry, so therefore can't possibly do anything till he's eaten. It doesn't matter that I might go without my lunch or dinner because something has to be done or the children need to be somewhere! He can never listen nor multi-task nor remember. Pants and socks are every day left on the floor, just where he hops into the bed, but the washing bin is only a foot away.
Rosie, London, mum to Sean, 10 and Owen, 7

When I ask him to do something for me, he says, 'Yeah, I'll do it later' or 'I'll do it at some point, don't worry.' Then he completely forgets and when I remind him he says I am nagging him and tells me not to nag or he won't do it.
Anna, Newcastle upon Tyne, mum to Dylan, 5 and Alex, 1

So how do you keep your relationship steady through the crazy years of child-rearing?

A quick gardening lesson

A relationship isn't like a house that once built will stay standing without changing for years and years and if it gets a bit run down you can always invest some time and money in later. A relationship is a dynamic, living, changing thing. Can you think of your relationship for a moment as a plant? It needs a little daily care. A plant doesn't need to be touched and held all day, but it does need regular water, food, air and sunlight. It needs awareness that it is a living thing and it needs daily sustenance.

So how can we give our relationship (our plant) the best possible chance to live and grow and be healthy? The first step is accepting that your relationship does need a basic level of care. Tell yourself that you won't put it at the bottom of the heap to dig out later, but that your relationship is important and that you will give it time and attention.

Basic relationship maintenance

This section is not about exploring deep-seated issues or saving relationships that are already in serious trouble. It's simply about how to take good, basic daily care of your relationship.

1. Be appreciative

Develop the wonderful virtue of gratitude. Everyone loves to feel appreciated and it's a wonderful motivator. Even if you wash up six times a day, every day, when your partner does the washing up, take a moment to say, 'Thank you for that', or 'That was such a help', or 'I'm very grateful for that.' Resist adding a sarcastic comment, such as, 'Shame you don't do it more often', or 'Pity I had to ask', as that takes all the good out of it. Just say, 'Thank you' and mean it.

2. Make a connection

How often do you make eye contact with your partner? How often do you really listen when you ask, 'How was your day?' Are you usually conversing while one of you cooks, cleans, tends a child, reads a magazine or watches telly?

It doesn't take any extra time and very little extra effort, so take a moment to make a real connection with each other two or three times in a day – a moment when you know you are a team, a moment to acknowledge through gestures that you care about each other and that you know life is very busy but you are still united.

In the morning, maybe make eye contact for a five full seconds and say something like: 'We're doing well, aren't we?', or We've a lovely little family, haven't we?', or 'We'll look back on these as good times.' Have a quick kiss or hug or squeeze of the hand. Perhaps send him a text message during the day that doesn't involve a moan or a request to bring home milk: *'Just to say hi, hope your day is going well.'* Or slip something into his jacket pocket – a note, a bar of his favourite chocolate. Create a moment in time, a moment when a real connection passes between you.

3. Spend time together

It's not rocket science but spending time together is probably the hardest thing to do. Think of it as money in the bank. It strengthens your relationship so that if you hit a difficult patch you have something to fall back on. Can you arrange half an hour in the pub once a week or an early evening supper in a local restaurant or even a posh coffee in a nice local café? Have you tried all possible avenues for babysitters or is it easier to fall back on the fact that you haven't got grandparents living near-by? Of course, if you are breastfeeding or coping with very clingy children, then that might not make sense right now, so book a date at home instead.

Agree that at least once a week you'll find an hour when you both agree to switch off the telly. If you can plan ahead, add something nice to eat or drink (a bottle of sparkling wine, a takeaway, or something more imaginative like a picnic in front of the fire). If you are worried you won't have anything to talk about, maybe bring out some old photos of when you first met or your first holiday together.

If you can also build in five minutes every day to sit together and say a proper hello to each other, that's great relationship maintenance!

4. Mark the transition to home life

When you all get home and back together at the end of the day, make it a point to stop for ten or fifteen minutes for a cup of tea or a bottle of beer. You've had your heads in different places: your work, his work, your children's lives . . . and now it's the end of another busy day. Before you go into 'evening mode', which might involve cooking, baths, homework, tidying and preparing for tomorrow, allow a little oasis to develop, a time when you can all stop, take a deep breath and bring your heads and your hearts back into the family home.

5. Hold an amnesty

Sometimes it can be little things that really annoy you. It might be something so insignificant that the other person is completely unaware of it. If left, these little things can build up into great mountains of resentment. Rather than letting the pressure build until it blows up one day, try holding an amnesty.

Explain to your partner what an amnesty is and that you'd like to book one. Explain that this means you have some small thing that you want to get off your chest but don't want to row. The amnesty part means that you get to have your say without him feeling he is being criticised and needing to retaliate. And, of course, he gets to 'hand in his weapons' too!

Choose a time when neither of you is stressed. It's also best not to do this over drinks, as alcohol loosens your tongue a bit too much and you may end up sparking off a full-blown row. Then say, in a matter-of-fact way, that when he leaves his socks all over the place it gets you down. Or that he always leaves his stubble in the bathroom sink for you to clear up. Tell him that you realise it's a small thing and not important in the grand scheme of life, but that it helps to get these things off your chest and if he could be aware they bother you and start to pick up his socks or rinse out the stubble, then it would stop you from overreacting. The deal with an amnesty is that he isn't allowed to argue but must just say, 'OK'! Then it's his turn to say if anything is bothering him. Each of you is allowed one thing each and then it's over. End it with a smile, a kiss or a handshake – some positive gesture – and get back to normal.

6. Commit to your relationship

Maybe you are married, in which case you made a very formal commitment. Or maybe you planned a baby together, which is a very big commitment. You may have publicly made those commitments but you may not have made that commitment deep down inside yourself. Often we marry or have babies when we are emotionally quite young. We can't really understand all that stuff about 'for better and for worse' until we've been through some bad times. We don't quite get 'in sickness and in health' until we've had sickness in the home. And we didn't really have any idea how long 'until death do us part' actually is!

Many of us also have this idea that it is our partner's role to take care of us and to make us happy. Do we also take on board that our side of the bargain is to care for our partner? A quiet, mature form of commitment is saying to yourself something like: 'I love him and I place a high value on our life together, therefore I will give it my love, care and attention.' Or 'I have chosen to be in this relationship and I *choose now* to continue to be in it. I am 50 per cent responsible for the success of this relationship. I will do my part and my best to care for my partner and to help him to be happy.'

7. Apologise

Saying you're sorry does not mean losing the battle. Saying you're sorry is a strength, not a weakness. If you were at fault, be prepared to accept it. Even if you were partly at fault, if even less than half of it was your fault, try to offer your apologies first. Apologising can be the first building block of a great bridge. If you find it really, really hard to say sorry, could it be that you feel you are locked in a constant battle with your partner? The clue is in the title: 'partner'. Fighting each other is a waste of good energy that you could be spending elsewhere. It shouldn't be you two against each other – it should be you two against the world!

8. Don't let the sun go down on your anger

Such a hard one! Stomping off to bed cross and resentful can feel quite good. You get the last word. You make him think. You punish him. But we know it's not a good thing for any of us. Sleeping on these feelings allows them to sink into our subconscious and the residue hangs around for ages. Couple that with the fact that going to bed cross will also interrupt our beauty sleep, and resolving things starts to seem the sensible option.

Make it a simple rule that you'll go to bed friends. It might mean sorting something out, or being the first one to say sorry (see above). Or it might mean agreeing that you need to talk about this issue when you are both calmer or less stressed or have more time, so you'll put it on hold for now and stay friends in the meantime. Sometimes just a hug will do it. Chances are he doesn't want to fight either.

9. Praise him

The same psychology that tells us to reinforce positive behaviour in our children applies to adults, whether it is to motivate a workforce or a husband! We all need to hear that we are doing well and that we are successful and valued.

Every day, try to find one good thing about your partner and tell him. If he's playing with the children, you might say, 'You're so good at playing rough and tumble with them – they love it and that's something a dad does best.' Or 'You are so much better at helping them with their homework – you've got such patience.' It makes a lovely change from criticism and you'll both enjoy the positive atmosphere it creates.

10. Give gracefully

If your partner asks you for something, try doing it cheerfully rather than begrudgingly. Maybe it's making him a cup of tea, or maybe it's getting a letter posted – or something bigger, like taking the children to see his mother. As long as it's something acceptable to you, do it without a fuss. Occasionally do something nice and special without being asked.

11. Have a laugh

Often laughing is the first thing to go when a relationship is under strain – yes, even before sex (we rarely laugh out of duty). Life can be tough, but we can also take both life and ourselves too seriously at times. It can be a good life and we are the only people who can make ourselves enjoy it. Bring a bit of fun back into your relationship. Lighten up, crack a joke, make each other laugh!

Arguing

We all do it. Many a survey has asked what we fight about most and the Top Five always include, in varying order, the following issues:

1. Money
2. Sex
3. Children

4. Work
5. Family

Does that sound familiar? Would it surprise you if you were told that when you are fighting about money, you aren't really fighting about money? Or when you're arguing about sex, it's not just sex you are arguing about? Relationships are hugely complex and much more so when you bring children into the equation. The focal point of an argument is just the tip of the argument iceberg. What we are dealing with is a whole host of underlying issues.

Let's take, for example, a simple argument about money. Lucy is upset because her partner, Mark, has spent £200 on a new fishing rod. Lucy tells Mark he is selfish and putting his own needs above the children. She says she can think of many things they need more than a fishing rod and that he should have consulted her first. Hadn't they agreed to make joint decisions?

All her words might be about the fishing rod, but underneath there is lots of other stuff going on:

◆ Insecurity: Why does he want to spend all that time away from her, fishing ?
◆ Jealousy: He is able to have a life and still enjoy his hobbies while she is stuck at home.
◆ Vulnerability: They used to be equal. He is the main breadwinner now. Where does that leave her in terms of equality?
◆ Resentment: She never gets the time to do her own thing any more.

In another example, John meets an old friend on the way home from work and stops off for a couple of pints. He's an hour and a half late. He doesn't go out much, but Polly, his wife, reacts badly. She's been looking after the children all day, she says she's exhausted and he's so selfish and never pulls his weight. If we look a bit deeper, we find out that Polly's father regularly came home from work drunk and left her mother in tears. John's one visit to the pub stirs up a childhood full of worry and powerlessness. Her reaction has little to do with John's behaviour and everything to do with her own childhood experiences.

Every one of us comes to a relationship with emotional baggage from our past of one sort or another. Imagine for a moment that our emotional self looks like a pond. The water may look clear on the surface but at the bottom of every pond is mud – deep mud in some ponds, less in others. An argument, especially with your partner, who is probably the closest person to you in the world, is like taking a stick and stirring up the pond. It brings the mud to the surface and makes the whole pond look muddy and murky.

In order to resolve conflict and disagreement, we first need to know:

1. Why we are feeling what we are feeling
2. What it is we want to achieve
3. What a realistic and acceptable outcome would be for both parties

Back to the fishing example: if Lucy can understand that the reason she is so angry is not because of the £200 but because she feels resentful that she doesn't have a life of her own, then maybe she can start to work towards an agreement with Mark that gives him time off for fishing and her time off to do something of her own.

Resolving conflict without a fight

Arguing and fighting seldom have a successful outcome. In a fight, there may well be a winner and it may well be you. But there will also be a loser, which means at least one of you will be feeling upset, angry, battered and bruised, and probably resentful. If one partner is always the loser (i.e. there is one more dominant partner), then the danger is that the less strong partner either will withdraw and perhaps start to hide things or will be quietly, internally angry for a long time and then one day will simply have had enough and will leave the marriage over something that looks fairly small from the outside. As you are partners, you need to aim to have two winners. All successful negotiators will agree that the right outcome is a win–win situation – no losers.

Ask yourself:

How can I avoid conflict?

The next time you find yourself getting cross or upset with your partner about something, instead of challenging him straight away, try this: walk away. Sit down with a piece of paper and write down what it is that is annoying or upsetting you. Draw a circle around it and around the outside write how this makes you feel. Be as specific as you can; rather than 'unhappy', try words or phrases such as: 'I feel vulnerable, not needed, unimportant.' Think about other times in your life when you felt like this: with your parents as a child, with your friends as a teenager, in a previous relationship? Ask yourself: 'Am I mixing this issue up with other issues? Has this matter been a big stick in my muddy pond?'

Now go back to what it is you wanted to challenge your partner about. Can you separate that issue from all the emotion it has raised?

If you have carried out this exercise, you will now have two things to talk to your partner about:

1. The Stick (e.g. the fishing rod)

2. The Mud it stirred up (e.g. feeling resentful about having no time to yourself)

The stick is probably something that doesn't seem quite as big now. Deal with it by avoiding blame and criticism. Use phrases such as: 'I feel upset by . . .' rather than '*You make* me feel upset . . .' Ask for what you want as specifically as possible without high drama – tears, shouting, sulking. For example, 'Will you agree that before we make any major purchases/decisions we'll have a chat about it first?'

Now you have resolved the stick, you can look at the mud. The important thing here is that you don't let it have too much influence over your relationship. You also should decide whether it is something you need to resolve within your own self. It might be that being aware of it is enough, or it might be something that you realise will always be a negative painful emotion and one that needs to be dealt with by a professional counsellor. Your GP is a great place to start. Read Chapter 9, Beating the Blues, for more about counselling.

Serious problems

If your problems are much bigger than the normal day-to-day relationship issues most couples face, don't feel embarrassed about getting professional help. It doesn't mean you are a failure; it means your relationship is important enough for both of you to try to fix it.

Couple counselling – or marriage guidance – offers a series of counselling sessions attended by both of you along with a trained counsellor. This creates a place in your lives where each of you can speak openly about your thoughts, feelings and needs without being judged or criticised. The counsellor creates this safe place where you can both be heard and understood. The aim is to develop your ability to communicate without feeling threatened and thus being defensive.

Your understanding of each other will develop and through this understanding you can learn to accept each other, forgive each other, appreciate each other – and love each other. Start with Relate. You can chat a bit on the phone first. They are used to speaking to people in sensitive situations and will be kind and understanding.

Don't stick your head in the sand. If you feel there are real problems developing in your relationship, there is no harm in booking a few sessions to get things back on track. It's the 'prevention is better than a cure' argument. Living with a relationship that has gone off track is exhausting and will make you miserable. Life is so much easier when you are best friends again.

There is no right or wrong way to go about resolving issues that do crop up – everyone is different and every scenario is different. It is important not to lose sight of yourself. Surround yourself with the people who mean the most to you. Real friends will let you talk and talk and talk when you are ready to. Don't feel guilty: that is what friends are for, and you would do the same for them.

Try to remember that it is very rare one party is wholly to blame for anything. Even an affair doesn't always mean the end of a relationship, although a complete break from each other is often needed so that talking and conversations can happen when the hurt has died down. Both parties need to think about why things happened. Invariably not communicating is the number one reason that adultery takes place.

When there are children involved, we have to be grown-ups, no matter how hurt and angry we are. If you are at a stage where you can't be grown up in front of them, then don't have conversations when they are around. Honesty is best, though be age appropriate, of course. A child doesn't need to know that Daddy is having sex with his secretary, but he can know that Daddy has hurt Mummy very much and that she is very upset, but he still wants to spend lots of time with his child, who is hugely important to him.

If you get to a stage where reconciliation is impossible, think about Family Mediation, for families in the process of separation or divorce. It may be the last thing you feel like, but sessions can help you deal with anger and bitterness. And if children are involved this can only be a good thing. If the children are old enough, and your counsellor agrees, they can also attend some or all of the sessions. The example we set our children will shape how they experience their relationships. Start with the National Family Mediation charity at www.nfm.org.uk

Physical violence or emotional abuse

We have looked at how we can do our best to make our relationship work and about how it is rarely all one person's fault; we take equal share for both good times and bad. However, there is an exception: physical or emotional abuse is *never* your fault in any way. It is *never* acceptable and can rarely be put right with an apology, however genuine and heartfelt.

At Netmums, we have talked to a shocking number of mums who are experiencing domestic abuse without having any idea that they are experiencing abuse. They may feel they haven't tried hard enough, have been lacking in some way as a wife or mother or that their partner was having such a hard time they needed to make allowances. It has often been the case that only by pointing out the definition of domestic violence to them that they were able to recognise it as such.

Here is a list from Women's Aid to help you to recognise if you are in an abusive relationship. Are you being subjected to:

◆ Destructive criticism and verbal abuse: shouting, mocking, accusing, name calling, verbally threatening.

- Pressure tactics: sulking; threats to withhold money, disconnect the telephone, take the car away, commit suicide, take the children away, report you to welfare agencies unless you comply with his demands regarding bringing up the children; lying to your friends and family about you; telling you that you have no choice in any decisions.

- Disrespect: persistently putting you down in front of other people; not listening or responding when you talk; interrupting your telephone calls; taking money from your purse without asking; refusing to help with childcare or housework.

- Breaking trust: lying to you; withholding information from you; being jealous; having other relationships; breaking promises and shared agreements.

- Isolation: monitoring or blocking your telephone calls; telling you where you can and cannot go; preventing you from seeing friends and relatives.

- Harassment: following you; checking up on you; opening your mail; repeatedly checking to see who has telephoned you; embarrassing you in public.

- Threats: making angry gestures; using physical size to intimidate; shouting you down; destroying your possessions; breaking things; punching walls; wielding a knife or a gun; threatening to kill or harm you and the children.

- Sexual violence: using force, threats or intimidation to make you perform sexual acts; having sex with you when you don't want to have sex; any degrading treatment based on your sexual orientation.

- Physical violence: punching; slapping; hitting; biting; pinching; kicking; pulling hair out; pushing; shoving; burning; strangling.

- Denial: saying the abuse doesn't happen; saying you caused the abusive behaviour; being publicly gentle and patient; crying and begging for forgiveness; saying it will never happen again.

If any of this seems familiar, then you are probably in an abusive relationship. This is not your fault and not something over which you have control. Your partner may be emotionally damaged himself or mentally ill, but you cannot help him by accepting the abuse. There is rarely an isolated incident and the statistics say that the abuse will escalate and get worse.

The women at Women's Aid are wonderful. You can call for a chat, anonymously if you prefer. Also, their website is very informative and has a copy of *The Survivors' Handbook*. There is a button on the website that you can press to remove any history or trail of you having visited that site. You can call the twenty-four-hour domestic violence helpline on 0808 2000 247, or visit the Women's Aid website at www.womensaid.org.uk

5 To Work or Not to Work?

Oh, the guilt! When you are at work, you feel guilty about not being with your child, and when you are with your child, you feel guilty about not being at work. And you feel guilty wherever you are if you so much as stop for a coffee break, as there is surely something more important to do and if you work a bit harder or a bit faster you might catch up by the weekend! Your quality of life is poor and time for yourself is non-existent. You pass by your husband (remember him?) on the stairs and you grunt instructions at each other. Occasionally you both stop and realise how crazy your lives have become. You both agree: there must be another way. So you talk over the options, go round in circles and find yourselves back where you started. You sigh, pick yourselves up and get on with it. Next year things will be easier. And we'll buy that lottery ticket on Saturday . . . you never know!

How things have changed! In the sixties it was all about equality – about giving women a chance, about giving women a *choice*. We got our choice. Then the debate raged about whether mothers should stay at home with their children or whether they should be able to have fulfilling careers. But somewhere things got a bit mixed up and somehow we haven't ended up with the choices we expected to have. How ironic that the great majority of mothers now have little choice: they simply have to work to make ends meet.

This chapter is about re-examining your choices, widening the options and finding the best possible balance for you and your family within the existing constraints.

Everything changes

When you asked yourselves if you could afford a baby or when you found out you were pregnant, at some point you may have sat down with your calculator to work it all out, but you probably accepted that you would have a bit less money. After all, even if you planned to go back to full-time work, childcare would have to be paid for. So you were prepared for certain lifestyle changes. Most mums, however, are completely unprepared for the complex emotional issues they have to face and we seldom factor these into our carefully laid plans.

Many of us are unprepared for the deep, overpowering love and protective instinct we feel for our babies. Or the tug of love and guilt that makes going back to work seem like crossing a field of unexploded and unmarked mines. Maternity leave, which in pregnancy seemed to stretch endlessly into the future, now seems a ridiculously short few months. The local nursery full of nice sensible childminders you visited and had down as 'option number one' suddenly seems a noisy and overwhelming institution full of strangers. The concept of working four days a week had seemed the perfect solution, as you would have three days with your child; suddenly you see it as four endless days without your child. Having your mother-in-law look after the baby means keeping it in the family and knowing your child is with someone who loves him; you just hadn't expected to feel so jealous. Everything has changed. You are looking at the world through different eyes: the eyes of a mother.

No perfect solution

The first barrier to overcome is to accept that there is not going to be a perfect solution. Full-time working mums miss the time with their children. Part-time working mums feel they have a foot in both camps but are not quite fully part of either. Stay-at-home mums often feel bored, undervalued and lonely. Simply by accepting that there is no perfect answer, you will have made significant progress towards feeling happier about your situation.

What are the options?
- Going back to the same job full time
- Going back to the same job part time
- Finding a different part-time job
- Working from home for an employer
- Becoming self-employed
- Giving up work to become a full-time mum

First of all, it is hugely helpful to realise that none of the decisions you make now are for ever. In fact, your working or not working situation may change many times over the years when you have very young children.

Ask yourself:

What is best for you and your family right now?

Helen was a personal assistant to a company director. After her six months' maternity leave when her first child was born, she found a nursery place for the child and went back to full-time work. Two years later, when her second baby arrived, they found the nursery runs, cost of childcare and general logistics too daunting, so the family looked again at their options and decided that Helen would stay at home with the children. Only a year later, their first child started school and Helen found she had more time and energy, so she started working from home as an Avon lady. This brought in a small income but enough for a few luxuries and gave Helen something just for herself. When her second child started school, Helen was able to take a job from 9am to 3pm in the office of a local school and, a couple of years later, they felt the children were ready for an after-school club, so Helen went back to full-time work.

So, in this case, Helen combined a mixture of options, with time spent:

– on maternity leave
– as a full-time working mum
– as a self-employed mum
– as a part-time working mum
– and back to full-time working mum.

Helen went full circle in eight years. The children had the best care possible, the family didn't overstretch themselves and Helen got to spend some time with her children when they were very young.

Full-time working mums – which one are you?

'I want to work full time.'

You worked hard at school, went to university, got a good degree, worked hard at your job and enjoyed a fulfilling and rewarding career. You've chosen to go back to work full time. Good for you. It is often indecision and lack of direction that makes us unhappy, whereas you have weighed up the options and made a decision.

Check out the happiness tips for full-time working mums on p. 139.

'I must work full time or it will affect my career.'

You've worked your way up the career ladder and you're on the fast track to success. If you bail out now, there are plenty of younger women (and men) only too happy to leap into your position and you don't want to give up your place to them. If you feel like this, then this is not the same as *wanting* to work. This is being scared not to. It feels like you need to choose: your career or your children; whereas a mum who wants to work finds a way for children and job to co-exist. Are you basing your life choices on the right motivation? You may need to ask yourself some hard questions:

- Do you need the status and power your job gives you?
- How is your self-esteem? What do you really think of yourself without your job?
- Why are you afraid to take some time out? What is that fear based on? Is it insecurity?

If you do decide to take time out for a few years, then could you spend some of that time brushing up on the skills you feel you are lacking? If you are somewhere between thirty and forty years of age, you may feel that if you bail out now you'll never get back in – at least, not at this level. And that is probably true if you are a model or maybe an actress. The rest of us are probably going to carry on working until we are sixty-five, or even later if we want to or have to. So, even if you take a five-year career break, and then spend a couple of years covering old ground while you catch up with your previous position, that still leaves you around thirty good working years! And the added balance and maturity you'll have gained during your years as a mother will give you something those thrusting twenty-five year olds don't have. Only you can make the right decision for you. Go with your heart not your head and the rest will fall into place.

'I have to work full time.'

In a Netmums' survey of full-time working mums, 50 per cent said they were unhappy working full time but had absolutely no other option because they needed their full-time salary.

It is tough to leave your children to go to work, especially if you are going to a fairly unsatisfying job rather than a fulfilling career. It is heartbreaking to hear the many stories of mums just returned from maternity leave who have had to tear themselves away from their child and can be found crying in the ladies' loo mid-morning. But these mums do adjust, and they do cope, as you will. Comfort yourself with the knowledge that children need very little to thrive in materialistic terms. What they do need is security and love, and you can (and do) provide these in abundance. Be proud of yourself: you are doing your best. If you are desperately unhappy, consider whether it is worth looking at your family budget with a fresh eye. The exercise on pp. 161–2 is designed to help you to do that and to reassess your priorities. Could it be that there is another solution?

'I work full time because I feel that my job is not a job that can be done part time. My employer wouldn't consider it.'

Maybe you've asked and been refused part-time work, or you feel it is a waste of time to ask. The law now says that parents have a right to request part-time work from their employers. However, employers also have the right to refuse, so, if you would like to reduce your hours at work, it is worth presenting your case as professionally and in as well-thought-out a manner as possible. Consider a solution that would work not only for you but also for the team or department you work in *and* for your boss and the company as a whole, and present that as a possibility. Rather than presenting your request as a request, consider presenting it as a solution. Give your employer something that is easy to say 'Yes' to.

These are the options you might request:

1. **Part-time working:** This is defined as anything below the standard working week.
2. **Flexi-time:** You work a guaranteed fixed number of hours per week or month but can take banked hours as flexible leave.
3. **Job-sharing:** The job is split so you share it with someone else.
4. **Term-time working:** This allows you to be in a permanent full- or part-time job while taking unpaid leave during agreed school holidays. Your pay may be averaged out over the year.
5. **School-hours working:** You work during school hours only.
6. **Compressed hours:** You work more hours each day, but fewer days of the week.
7. **V-time** (voluntary reduction in hours): V-time allows you to reduce your time at work by an agreed period.
8. **Working from home:** You can work from home all or part of the week. This can be done if you have older children, but don't expect to be able to work and look after a baby or young child at the same time.

If you believe your job can be done as a job share, type out your request and present it professionally to your boss, explaining how it would work, who would work what hours, who would cover what duties, how handovers would be managed and the advantages (two energetic employees rather than one tired one!). Ask a friend or colleague to help you set out the arguments and to quiz you on how it would work. Maybe even find someone who would like to job share with you or tell the boss you will take on the task of finding someone for him to interview. Give the request to your line manager but consider copying it to your managing director or the head of human resources.

Requests for part-time work

The law says:

♦ If you have a child under six, and have been working with an employer for at least 26 weeks, you can request flexible work, which means you could change days, working hours or your place of work.

♦ You must put your request in writing.

♦ Your employer must hold a meeting with you within 28 days of receiving your letter, and must give you their decision within 14 days of that meeting.

♦ You are also entitled to have a meeting with your employer to discuss your request, and you can take someone with you, such as a friend or a trade union representative. An employer must consider a request for flexible working seriously and can refuse only for one of the following 'business reasons':
  – The burden of additional costs
  – The detrimental effect on the ability to meet customer demand
  – The detrimental effect on quality
  – If the employer is unable to recruit additional staff
  – If there is not enough work during the period the employee wants to work
  – If there are planned structural changes.

If you think your employer did not follow the correct procedure, or took a decision for an invalid reason, you can appeal. If unsuccessful, you may make a complaint to an employment tribunal, or take it up as a case of sex discrimination. The employment tribunal will award a maximum of eight weeks' pay in compensation, up to £270 per week. Awards for sex discrimination are not limited. Take advice on your options and the most appropriate action.

Eight happiness tips for full-time working mums

1. Get the best possible childcare you can afford (see Chapter 6, Who's Caring for Your Kids?).
2. Ditch the guilt. As far as is humanly (or maternally) possible, try to stop feeling guilty. If you have weighed up all the options and looked at all the facts, then hold your head high and stand by your decision. You have made the best decision possible for you and for your family at this time. If you feel confident in your decision, then others will also accept that it was the best one for your family.
3. When you are there, be there! When you get in from work, get down to your children's level and truly be with them – not with one eye on the washing machine and one ear on the phone. For a short time, give them your undivided attention.
4. Don't try to catch up with your children's day by firing lots of questions at them – you won't be much the wiser at the end of your interrogation. Get the information you crave from your childminder, nursery or nanny. Ask them to keep a record book if it helps you to catch up with the children's day. When you are with your children, just be with them, play a gentle game with them, sit and read to them or sit near them as they play. Have a

calm and peaceful atmosphere and you may find little golden nuggets of information being passed your way as thoughts cross their little minds.

5. Look after yourself. We don't believe in supermums. We're all human – just mums. You can't manage a full-time career, run a house and all that goes with it, and be a perfect mum and a fabulous wife without something cracking somewhere. See Chapter 8, What About Me?, which relates as much, if not more, to full-time working mums as it does to stay-at-home mums.

6. If money allows, delegate as much household work as possible: get a cleaner and send out the ironing. Some women might feel slightly shamed not to be looking after their own home, but you already have a job and you work hard at it. You are also a mum, so if it's a toss-up between spending your evenings cleaning, hoovering and ironing or spending time with your children, then it's no contest! Contract out as much as you can possibly afford. Most of the local cleaners and ironing services are done or run by mums looking to make a little extra money, so you're also helping mum-kind.

7. Stop every so often to review your life, your goals and ambitions. Be careful that you're not so busy rushing along that you've forgotten what your destination is.

8. Don't buy your child 'stuff' through guilt to make yourself feel better or to compensate for not being there. It won't make you or your child any happier and it sends out all the wrong signals. Instead, make a date with your child – even if it's just once a week – when you do something lovely together: swimming or horse-riding or jumping in muddy puddles. That's what your child wants: to see you laughing and having fun with him.

Ask the Netmums:

Do you work full time? If so, is it by choice or necessity?

I work full time and almost always have done. I wouldn't say I have always needed to, but now if I didn't, our family income would be halved, and we would have to make some serious changes, as the mortgage and associated costs would swallow up around half of my other half's salary.

My kids are eight and five, and I went back to work as soon as my paid maternity leave ran out (after eighteen weeks, both times). I now work flexible hours 9.30–5.30 so I can take the kids to school each day. It was definitely harder emotionally going back after my second, as I had more of an idea of what I might miss out on by being at work, so I did a few weeks of part time to adjust back to working.

As the kids have got older, it has got a lot harder. Schools, in particular, don't make it easy on working parents, as there is always something going on that you are invited to attend and you feel really guilty if your little one says, 'Are you coming, Mummy? All my friends' mummies will be there.' My other half works thirty-odd miles away, travelling by train, so he can't easily share the load (two harvest festival assemblies in one week, book fairs, different parents' evenings for different classes at the same school, concerts and plays, reading workshops – the list gets longer all the time). There is more homework to fit in when you finally get home and pick the kids up (I have two lots of reading every night, two lots of spellings, one lot of maths and one lot of literacy homework every week, recorder practice every week plus occasional homework for my youngest). A further challenge is out-of-school activities. Most of these don't fit around working, so I need to find ways to accommodate such things as swimming lessons on Saturday mornings (the weekday slots are 4–6pm), to leave work early (no lunch break) to get to Beavers on time (5.45–7.15pm), to try to get music lessons after 6pm (still trying), and to beg favours from other mums to get to parties. We also try to have an active family life at weekends (caravanning at weekends and holidays, walking in the Peak District), so we don't have much time when we stop and do nothing . . . TV is generally something we watch when doing the ironing!

To anybody who is trying to decide if they will go back: if you don't need to, think long and hard about whether you want to. I need a full-time salary for part-time hours and then I'll have it cracked!

Katrina, Doncaster, mum to two children aged 8 and 5

I work out of choice. I work in a college, so I work only during term time. To be honest, I go stir crazy during the holidays and actually look forward to going back to work, although we have been back three weeks now and I'm looking forward to the next holiday. I think working term time gives me the best of both worlds.

Alison, Kent, mum to two daughters aged 16 and 4

I feel like I have the best of both worlds! I have registered as a childminder since having Daniel, and look after three other children now. Although I am working full time, Daniel is with me all the time too. I have always worked in childcare, so it just seemed a natural progression when Daniel came along. As I have spent the last twenty years looking after other people's children, it would be mad for

me to leave him with someone else while I went out to work.
Jayne, Leigh-on-Sea, mum to Daniel, 17 months

I work full time but it's on a basis of five days on, five days off
. . . twelve-hour shifts. I do this out of choice, because I want
to have the money to provide my two children with the stuff
they want and to live comfortably. The shifts I do have given
me more time with my children than a nine to five job would
with just weekends off.

Some shifts I work are nights, so I get to spend time with
them in the day and am at work when they're in bed and
home in time to take them to school in the morning, I just
live on little sleep! It works very well in our household; the
children are never without and they have either me or
Daddy here.
Jemma, Carshalton, mum to Jack, 8 and Alex, 2

I went back to work full time when my daughter was thirteen
weeks old. It was mentally very difficult for me. Thankfully we
have a great childminder who was one of our friends before
we had our daughter, and she always gives her loads of
kisses and cuddles and treats her like one of her own. Both
me and my husband travel abroad for two to four days at
a time and we have no family locally. People ask me how
we did it (our daughter is now three) and I just say, 'It's mind
over matter.' For the first year I thought I would collapse with
exhaustion but it's fairly manageable now. As soon as we
come home from work every day we spend two hours
playing with our daughter and don't do any chores until she
goes to bed. We also spend most of our weekends doing
things with her. She seems a happy, balanced child – so far,
so good. Basically, I would work less if I could but I can't find

any managerial jobs on a part-time basis that also pay a decent salary.

Patricia, Bristol, mum to Sonia, 3

I have worked full time since Troy was nine months old. I chose to go back to work (a different job from the one I did before Troy) and I love my job to bits; it's fantastic. My hubby's family help out with childcare and Troy also goes to a childminder, which has done him the world of good. He has become a proper toddler now, which we love. It is hard being a working mum with chores on top, but I love my time at work and enjoy Troy more. I am also lucky that hubby's parents help us out so much. I could not be a stay-at-home mum and think that mums who do stay at home do a wonderful job. Each to her own; you should do what you think is right for you, no one else. At times being a full-time working mum is hard and sometimes I think, 'Why do I bother?', but I know it's the right situation for me and my family. Troy does not miss out on anything, even if it means doing it in the evening or taking a day off. Be prepared for hard work, but don't let people make you feel guilty for doing what you want to do in life. It is better to be happy than miserable.

Sarah, Leicestershire, mum to Troy, 2

I work full time because I have to. Flexi-working has been great, although sometimes I feel I miss so much in their growing up. I found it really difficult to adjust from maternity leave to working full time but now I have accepted it because I have to – otherwise we would have no home or money, especially with twins!

Joanne, Newtownabbey, Northern Ireland, mum to twin boys, Johnathan and Aidan, 3

I'm a single mum and I work full time, but it's shift work, which does have its good side, as my daughter is often in bed when I'm working some of my hours. The problem now is, because she has started school, some days I see her for half an hour in the morning and don't see her until I collect her from school the next day.

This brings tears to my eyes just thinking about it, as given half a chance I'd be a stay-at-home mum spending time with my child.

Louise, Newcastle-under-Lyme, mum to Grace, 3

Part-time work

In recent Netmums research of 4,000 mums, we discovered that only 12 per cent of those mums working full-time were entirely happy with the situation. By contrast, 62 per cent of those working part-time were happy with their situation. So in the pursuit of happiness, part-time work does seem to be an option worth serious exploration. The down side is that you can feel not quite part of the office culture and not quite accepted by the full-time mums.

Five happiness tips for part-time working mums

1. Make friends with other mums. Have a routine of scheduled activities with other mums and children during your days off from work. Find a toddler group that is open on your day off or join a mother and child swimming or singing class.
2. Don't disengage from all work social events. It is hard to find time and energy, and you'll want to spend time with your family, but do try to join in the occasional after-work drinks. To a large extent your well-being and happiness come from being a part of

things, feeling included and accepted. Part-time workers often feel part of nothing.

3. Remember employers must, by law, treat part-time workers the same as full timers. You are entitled to the same training, holidays, salary and perks (pro rata, of course) as your full-time colleagues.

4. Don't feel guilty about leaving the office earlier than everyone else or for not being there on your days off. You work hard when you are there and you are being paid only for the hours that you do. Your childless colleagues might find it hard to understand but the higher you hold your head and the less you apologise for it, the more normal and acceptable you will make it seem.

5. You should not feel guilty for what you don't do at home while you are at work. Remember you have two *part-time* jobs: at work and at home. Don't try to do both full time or you'll be trying to squeeze 80 hours into 40. And you are a mum all the time, which means busy evenings, disturbed nights, family weekends. Be reasonable with yourself about how much it is sensible for any one person to try to achieve. Read Chapter 8, What About Me?

Ask the Netmums:

Do you work part time?

I work part time. It has been really hard to find something, but I was determined. The employer I was with when I had my son did offer me a part-time job but it was totally impractical. I would have had to go in every day and would have lost all the benefits that went with the full-time post, so I quit. I now work a bit from home and a bit in an office. The pay is OK but I'm not on a proper contract. I am still applying for part-time jobs on the rare occasions I see them advertised and hope to find something with reasonable

pay and benefits; they exist but there is stiff competition. I would love not to work at all but we need the money.
Camilla, Harrow, mum to Lukas, 19 months

I'm mum to three little ones, and currently on maternity leave from my part-time job of fifteen hours a week. I have asked to go back ten hours a week during school hours and they have agreed. I have had my share of part-time jobs since leaving full-time work and can honestly say it has always been hard to find suitable jobs, particularly when my eldest started school. I cannot fault my employers at all and they are very flexible when it comes to the little ones.
Karen, Wellingborough, Northamptonshire, mum to Hannah, 6, Gemma, 3 and Ruby, 11 months

I work part time delivering parcels for a catalogue company. It's the sort of job that fits in totally well with having a young child, as when she is with you, you just put her in the car along with the parcels and off you go. Total flexibility with hours – great. I just enquired and forgot all about it until I was contacted by my manager. It seemed to fit in really well and that was almost three years ago.
Ruth, Manchester, mum to Madelaine, 4

My employer allowed me back two days a week after being there full time for a few years. My son is two and a half and I now work two days a week as part of a job share. I also do Avon as well.
Tricia, Hertfordshire, mum to Jack, 2

I was made redundant three days after telling my employer I was pregnant! In the end, I started mystery shopping [covertly assessing staff and facilities so that a company can improve on the service it offers] and now am also a team leader for Usborne Books – both working from home. It means I can spend time with my toddler, and when I do need to go out to work, I only take on things where he can come too.

Tracey, Stockton-on-Tees, mum to Alexander, 20 months

I requested to go back part time and was told that this wasn't acceptable. So I came up with another plan – to do a job share. Luckily, an old colleague decided she could do with the hours and we got the perfect working arrangement: she works Monday to Wednesday (mornings) and I work Wednesday to Friday. It suits us both fine, and I've still got a handle on my career without being swamped.

June, East Lothian, mum to Eva, 2

I work part time, sixteen hours a week. I love my job as it's a bit of free time for me and Cameron loves going to nursery! I was originally looking for more hours, but this job was all that was available at the time. It has now turned out to be the perfect job for my circumstances – just enough hours to get working tax credit but not too many hours so I don't feel guilty about leaving Cameron at nursery too much! The time is perfect too: I work 2.30 till 5.30 every day. I can get everything done in the day and then head off to work, come home and spend some time with Cam before bedtime!

Amy, Grantham, mum to Cameron, 17 months

I have just found a job working Monday, Tuesday and Wednesday 8am–1pm and every fourth Saturday. While looking for this job though, I must have applied for over fifty

jobs in six weeks . . . with only four replies and two interviews. It's hard finding a part-time job.
Caroline, Wakefield, mum to James, 2

I work three days a week and find it a welcome break! It is the best of both worlds: I get to spend time with my kids but still have time when I am 'me' and not somebody's mum. It is also nice to have time off from thinking what you are going to do in the next fifteen minutes, especially when it is raining! I am lucky that my employers are very accommodating in trying to enable employees to work the hours that they want when they return following maternity leave. I think everyone should work a three-day week; there is something psychologically satisfying about knowing you are away from work more than you are there!
Emma, Pontefract, mum to Max, 2 and Tobias, 3 months

I work part time with two jobs. I work in a bar on a casual basis, and I also do waitressing two shifts a week. I don't earn a lot of money but it all helps at the end of the day. Because I work evenings and weekends, my husband looks after the kids and puts them to bed, so we have no childcare costs. I like my jobs, but there is a bit of a stigma attached – the 'Oh, you're just a barmaid' kind of thing. But I'm at home during the day with my toddler, which I really enjoy.
Tina, Kent, mum to Daisy, 2

I have four children and I work part time as a childminder. I started when my third child was two. It fits in really well around my kids!
Lisa, St Neots, mum to Andrew, 12, Emma, 9, Mathew, 7 and Adam, 2

I work for a local authority and I have found that they are very willing to consider part-time/job share/term-time-only working. I work four days (30 hours); in my office there are other people working four days (20 hours), three days (18 hours), etc.

I applied for the post, which was advertised as full time, and at interview told them I would only be able to work four days as I have a young son and want to have a good work/home life balance. To be honest, I thought if they didn't let me work four days I wouldn't have wanted the job anyway and thus for me it was something I would not compromise on. I was certain when I told them and I think this ensured we were all clear on what I would work, so there was no confusion when I was offered the job. I didn't write on the application form that I couldn't do full time, as I wanted to have my chance to dazzle (!) at interview before they ruled me out for that small reason.

So far working part time hasn't stopped me getting the last two jobs I've applied for – this permanent one and my previous temporary one. The scary bit is once you start the job and realise they expect the same amount of work as a full-timer – but that's a different issue! My childcare costs a fortune but for me it is worth it as I enjoy my job most of the time and get a buzz out of the work environment.
Anna, Maidstone, mum to Ben, 3

I have been working for the same company for eighteen years since leaving school. After having my first daughter, who is now six, I returned full time, as I was lucky to have a wonderful mum who looked after her. However, after having my second daughter, I felt it would be too much for my mum, plus I wanted to be able to take my eldest to school some days.

I mentioned to my boss before going on maternity leave about returning part time and she gave me a form to fill in which is standard practice for our company. I could say what days I wanted to work, etc., so I chose Monday to Wednesday usual office hours of 8.30 to 4pm. I am home by 5, so I still have the evenings with the girls. All my benefits are still the same, though some are pro rata, which is only fair. To be honest I would not work if we could afford it, probably like a lot of people, but I do find myself going to work on a Monday for a rest and a sit down! Won't tell the boss that, though!

Joanna, Dagenham, mum of kids aged 6 and 2

Before having the children, I worked full time as a solicitor, usually between forty and fifty hours a week. After having my son, I went back four days a week, 8am–6pm, but found that I was doing the same amount as I was doing before, just in less time, so I was bringing work home with me. When I fell pregnant again, I dropped my hours to 9am–4pm and tried to put my foot down about the extra work (I was getting paid only for the hours I was in the office, so I didn't see why I should do the extra). But after my daughter was born, I realised going back wouldn't work, plus the costs of childcare places for two children under two was crazy!

I now work from home selling children's books, and have no childcare costs, as the children come with me, so financially I'm actually better off than I was before. But no matter how hard I found my last job, it was a breeze compared to working from home and looking after two toddlers! At least I can be here to see them grow up, so I guess there are pros and cons to everything.

Stephanie, Harrogate, mum of two aged 3 and 20 months

Starting your own business

Women are amazingly creative and resourceful. When faced with a challenge like how to balance the household finances with looking after a toddler and a new baby, we can come up with an amazing array of ideas and options. If you don't want to work full time and can't find a suitable part-time job but can't quite afford to stay at home, then this section offers some alternatives. It's not about getting rich; it's about topping up the monthly budget by a few hundred pounds and achieving the best balance we can. Have you ever thought about doing your own thing and setting up your own small local business? Most successful entrepreneurs will say that the difference between them and others is that they actually did it. They didn't just think about it, or talk about it, or leave it until 'one day' – they made a start.

1. The idea

First of all you need your idea. What is it you will sell? Is it a *product* (something you make or buy in and sell on) or a *service* (something you can do for others)?

Here are a few ideas to start you thinking:

Products

Have you ever had a good idea for a new product aimed at mums and families? Do you make jewellery, or knit unusual but gorgeous tops? Do you design T-shirts? You could set up a little local business making and selling your work through local playgroups, craft fairs, school fêtes and home parties.

Household services

There is always a demand for cleaners and ironing services (particularly those that pick up and drop off). Again, local professional companies often have vacancies, or you could start small, offering the service through local nurseries.

Children's parties

Kids' parties are big business these days, with many mums too tired or busy at work to have time to do all their own planning, catering and entertainment. You could offer catering for children's parties, supply party bags or provide home-made themed birthday cakes. Children's party entertainers are often mums who are outgoing, enjoy being with children, like being on stage and have learned some good magic tricks.

Classes

Do you have a skill, or a special talent that you do well and enjoy? Netmums comes across lovely successful independent pre-school groups all over the country run by ordinary mums with a skill or interest in something. Dance, gym, music, art, cooking for kids . . . any of these make lovely pre-school groups for mums and tots. If you have lots of energy, a love of children and an interest or aptitude for music, dance, PE, or teaching maths or English, this could be a way to combine your skills with a balanced life.

Don't forget the mums! You could teach a small cookery, drawing, language, computing, music or gardening class. Many mums don't want to go to 'evening classes' but would love to meet up in a small group of four or five mums to learn a new skill while making friends – and they'd pay for it too.

2. The market

Once you know what you are going to sell – whether it's a service or a product – it is crucial you know who will want to buy it. Without a market, your business will fail, so find out everything you can. Start by thinking about whom you are targeting. Is it other mums? Are they local mums or mums all over the country?

Now look at your competitors. Are there other people around selling similar things? Is there room for both of you? What is different about what you will be doing and how will you persuade people to come to you instead of going to someone who is already established?

How will you reach your market?

Now you need to think about how you will market your service or product. It may be that there are some people who are easy to reach (family and friends might be your starting point), but as your business grows how will you get through to new customers? Advertising in the local paper can be costly and not always effective, so think about where your customers go and how you can tell them about your product or service.

Some ideas for local marketing:

- Think about how much time you've spent in doctors' waiting rooms staring at the walls. You'll need to be very nice to the receptionists, but if you are offering something useful many will be happy to pin a notice up for you.
- Do the rounds of the local mother and toddler groups. Ask the organisers if you can give out some leaflets or show some samples.
- Stand outside local schools at picking-up time and hand out leaflets, or ask the schools if they will put something in the children's book bags.
- Many pre-schools will agree to let you set up a little table or stall selling your products in return for a small percentage of sales (offer them 10 per cent).
- Look for local magazines aimed at families: it can be cheaper and more targeted.

3. The money

Now think about what your business needs to succeed. As you are working out the prices for your products or services, you must make sure you build in all your business costs. Think through how much stock, materials or equipment you will require and how much money you will need to spend on advertising. Remember that you might need help from an accountant at least once a year, so be sure you build in that cost too. Do a cash-flow forecast: work out how much you are spending to get the business set up and to buy stock in, and calculate the costs you will have to carry until you start to make some money back. Can you carry those costs for long enough? If you can, look at what you expect to happen over the next twelve months and work out what you need to do to break even as well as the turnover that you hope to achieve to make a profit. If you think you will have to find some money to help get the business off the ground, how much will you need?

What happens if your business does better or worse than expected? How will you manage the flow of work?

There are legal requirements if you are running a company and you should set aside time to make sure you are aware of them. Do you need insurance? What taxes will you have to pay? What accounting records (money in and money out) will you keep?

4. Your business plan

Now write it all up. This is called your business plan. Make sure you start by clearly describing what you are doing and why it will appeal to others. Whether you need funding or not, it is a good idea to take it to talk to your small business adviser locally. Business Link, businesslink.gov.uk, the national business advice service, provides some great practical advice and has lots of interactive tools to help you get organised. There's also a postcode search to help you find contact details for your local Business Link. Use it for advice and help with business plans, etc., or to access a wide network of business support organisations.

Direct selling

If you think you can sell locally, but aren't ready or able to start making your own product, you could opt for something called 'direct selling'. Remember the Avon lady? Well, she could be you! Or the Virgin cosmetics lady or the Body Shop at Home lady . . . Direct selling means you get the products straight from the company and sell them to the buyers without going through a shop. There are lots of reputable direct selling companies that you could work for (see Appendix I). You usually have to pay something towards your start-up kit, then they supply the products and you do your own local sales and marketing and you keep a percentage of whatever you sell. If you are incredibly dedicated and put in a lot of work, you can earn quite decent money, but if it's something you want to do part time, around the kids, then it can make you enough to top up your family income and make ends meet.

Franchising

If you'd like your own business but find the whole idea of planning and starting one a step too far, then buying a franchise could be for you. Franchising is a way of setting up in business for yourself but not on your own. You can buy a franchise to set up certain classes or groups in your area. These are the sorts of groups you may have attended yourself with your little ones: music, dance and gym classes. Of course, you could do something like this on your own, without buying a franchise, but with a franchise you will be using methods that have already been tried and tested by another company, called the franchisor.

You pay the franchisor for a package that gives you an exclusive 'territory' and allows you to use its brand name, methods of operation, technology or products for a certain period, say five years, on a renewable contract. Once accepted as a franchisee, you get technical and/or business training, operation manuals, often marketing help and sometimes accounting or other administration services. In return, you agree to run the business according to the franchisor's methods and standards. Each company varies in what they have to offer and what they require from you in return, so do check everything thoroughly before committing yourself to be sure that it is right for you.

The British Franchise Association (see p. 297) has details of available franchises and further information and advice about franchising. And there is a list at the back of this book about some franchises that are suitable for mums.

Childminding

Childminders work from their own homes. The beauty of this job is you can combine looking after your own children with looking after other people's. But do remember that professional childminders are exactly that: professionals. Childminding is not an informal arrangement to babysit someone else's child or an easy solution to how to bring in a bit of extra cash while minding your own child. You need to enjoy children – other people's as well as your own. Your child needs to be able to share you, his home and his toys with other children on a daily basis. And you need to be able to accept the daily extra mess and wear and tear that young children bring to your home. If you can accept all that, then you could be among the many mums who find childminding a happy solution to the problems of those early years.

To become a registered childminder, you have to go on an

introductory training course, which will cover topics such as child protection, child development and the business side of childminding. You will also need a current first-aid certificate that covers first aid for babies and young children. You must be registered with Ofsted and 'inspected' not just for safety in the home but to ensure that meals are properly planned and healthy and that you are equipped to educate as well as to 'play with' the children in your care.

To start, go to a local childminding pre-registration briefing session. This session tells you about becoming a childminder. Find out when the next session is by contacting your local Children's Information Service. You can find contact details by clicking on to www.childcarelink.gov.uk

Childminder start-up grants are available in both England and Wales. The grants, which are administered by Early Years Development and Childcare Partnerships (EYDCPs), are aimed at helping new childminders with the costs of setting up their childminding business. They provide money for toys, safety equipment, insurance, registration and inspection fees, National Childminding Association [NCMA] membership and tools of the trade. In 2006 the average sum awarded in England was £300.

Ask Yourself:

What can you do to improve your working situation?

Often, if we feel trapped in a situation, we lose our ability to look at the situation creatively. We also feel defensive and alone and forget to look at whether other people could help us in some way. If you are unhappy with your working situation or your work/life balance, try asking yourself these questions (using the SMART technique):

Specific: What exactly is the issue? It might be: 'Financially I have to work five days a week but I want to spend more time at home', or 'I'd like to spend more time at home but I find it so scary/boring/lonely that I'm working but for the wrong reasons.' What is it that is making you unhappy about the existing situation? Be honest with yourself: is there a deep-rooted feeling that you are hiding maybe even from yourself? Maybe you feel you want to be a full-time mum because you hate your job/boss. Or maybe you are working full time because you are scared to have less money and let go of material things you enjoy?

Measurable: What would be a good outcome? For example, it might be working a three-day week.

Achievable: Is that achievable? Often we say something is not achievable because we are afraid of the changes we would need to make to make it possible. If it were a life or death situation, would you find a way? What would or wouldn't matter if it really were a life or death situation?

Realistic: Is it realistic? It may be that being a full-time mum is not realistic but working a four-day week is. Or your present job may be very male-centred and your employer has never entertained the idea of part-time work. Could you be a pioneer and change that (for example, by going to the management) or is that not a battle you feel able to engage in? If the latter is the case, a change of employer may be the only option for achieving your goal.

Timely: When are you going to start?

If you are struggling to answer these questions, ask yourself: 'What is the smallest change I could make in my life that would bring me the biggest benefit?' And don't do it all on your own! Ask yourself: 'Who could help me to achieve this?'

Money, money, money

Money, of course, is the significant factor in your decision-making process. Whatever your thoughts, feelings and emotions, somehow the mortgage needs to be paid, the bills need to be taken care of, and the car needs to be kept on the road. Your family needs a basic income to cover your outgoings.

When men were the sole providers and most mums were full-time mums, the majority of young families didn't have much money. They certainly didn't have as much 'stuff' and they didn't have foreign holidays, two cars and wardrobes full of clothes. They didn't feel the need to furnish their homes with the latest decor in the most fashionable colour scheme nor to dress their children in designer clothes. Children played with simple, often home-made toys (yes, and your dad got an orange and some nuts in his stocking at Christmas and walked five miles to school in his bare feet). Things have changed: everybody has so much more now and it's very hard to be the one to make a stand and say 'materialism doesn't mean anything to me and we are going to be poor but happy' – and even if you are so noble, your husband might not be!

What to do is work out and agree what your needs are as a family. Research has shown time and again that once your basic needs are met (food, shelter, warmth), money and the stuff it buys do not contribute to levels of happiness. Indeed, in a study of lottery winners, although they seemed dramatically happier in the immediate aftermath of winning their prize, within two years their happiness levels had dropped back to the level they were before the win.

Ask yourself:

How much money do you need each month?

Get out the past six months' bank statements (one or two aren't enough to build a pattern). Write down all your monthly costs.

Fixed costs

Fixed costs are costs that must be paid, cannot be varied from month to month and cannot be avoided.
– Rent or mortgage
– Electricity
– Gas
– Phone (rental/line, not calls)
– Mobile phone (again, fixed monthly costs, not calls)
– Cable/satellite TV (do you really need it?)
– Broadband/internet connection
– Health insurance
– House/contents insurance
– Life insurance
– Car (loan/services/repairs/insurance)
– Debt payments (any debts/credit cards)
– Dentist (the annual family cost divided by twelve)

Variable costs

These are costs that you can control to an extent or vary

month on month. Write down your existing average spend.

– Car: petrol
– Food
– Clothes for your children
– Clothes for you and your partner
– Make-up/luxuries
– Hairdresser
– Presents for parties, family, etc.
– Presents for your children
– Entertainment for grown-ups: cinema, restaurants, takeaways, DVDs, etc.
– Entertainment for children: outings, farms, play centres, theme parks, lunches out
– Wine
– Holidays (total cost divided by twelve)
– Christmas (total cost divided by twelve)
– Childcare
– Other expenses?

Now can you see how much of your expenditure is luxury? Can you see where you could cut back? What could you quite happily do without? What could you just about do without?

Ask the Netmums:

What do you go without to be at home with your children?

We go without family holidays, as we can't afford to go anywhere, but we make up for this by taking day trips instead now and then . . . and personally I don't think a holiday is any better than a few well-spent days as a family at home. The kids go without expensive birthday parties; instead they have a great time with a family tea party and a few choice friends. This also goes for mum and dad. We don't go out for birthdays or anniversaries – or at least very rarely – and we don't go out for romantic evenings, as they have become unaffordable since we've had only one wage.

I don't think it really matters to us that we go without as such . . . we are happy together and we do things that make us happy. We've got our health and that's what's important to us, along with a roof over our heads and food in our tummies! Of course, it does get us down as parents sometimes when we have to say, 'No, you can't have a drink from the supermarket because there aren't enough pennies', or 'No, you can't have sweeties, a new toy, etc.' It is hard sometimes to see other families having great days out to these fantastic places like zoos or event type places that we just can't afford, but at the end of the day it's our love for our children and theirs for us that's important. I will eventually go back to work, but not until our family is complete and are all of an age that we won't need childcare.

Andrea, Leeds, mum to Mary Beth, 4 and Robert, 2

I have been a stay-at-home mum for four and a half years and, yes, we gave up a lot for me to do this, including my budding career. But my kids don't go without. Too much value today is placed on materialistic things and kids want, want, want and so do some parents. So we don't have three holidays abroad a year, we don't have the latest gadgets and my house is 'lived in' and needs much doing to it. But Mummy takes the children to school and picks them up every day. My kids are really happy. What more could you ask for?

Mary, Bristol, mum to Mollie, 4 and Connie, 19 months

I am not materialistic in any way. I love being a full-time stay-at-home mum and think it's the best job in the world. We don't do without as there is so much love and affection. We do lots as a family, my kids love me being there for them, our bills are paid and good food is on the table – what more can I ask?

Wendy, Harrow, mum to Glen, 6 and Greg, 5

I had worked for the same company for fifteen years and had worked hard to climb the career ladder and reached the position where I had a good salary, company car, private healthcare, pension, etc. We were able to enjoy a couple of holidays a year, as well as weekends away and meals out, and able to afford things we wanted as opposed to needed. As you can imagine, all this changed when I became a stay-at-home mum. We have one UK holiday on a budget, weekend breaks involve visiting family, an occasional takeaway has replaced the meals out and clothes tend to come from the supermarket or sales. I consider myself lucky in that we can afford to eat and pay our bills, but the time I spend with my son and the experiences I have a chance to share are far more precious than anything I now have to go without. I plan to go back to work when he's older, but gone are my days of living to work – I will now work to live.

Kathy, Leicester, mum to Jacob, 1

The best thing about having kids is sharing everything with them. Giving up work was tough but the best decision for me. I sacrifice things for myself so my kids can have whatever they need and I wouldn't change a thing.

Toni, Waltham Forest, mum to Chloe, 7 and Brandon, 2

'Giving up' a job sounds like the job was better than being a stay-at-home mum! I wake up every morning and thank God I'm not in that ghastly job and can revolve my life round kids (my own and the kids at their school, where I volunteer). I reckon my husband, who stays in his rotten job to bring home the salary, is the one who's sacrificing.
Katherine, London, mum to Rachel, 13 and Tom, 9

I have been 'home' for six years now, having given up a very well-paid and varied job. I don't particularly resent the loss of my own money, because my husband is generous and shares whatever is left over at the end of the month – and, of course, heavy-duty skirts and jeans don't really cost as much as the business suits and designer shoes! My hair is now long and I colour it myself instead of spending nearly £100 every six weeks and I no longer have manicures – not a problem at all.

What I really, really am starting to miss is the total loss of any personality. I am Ben and Imogen's mum and Julian's wife. I was taken to a business do the other day – talk about the 'little woman'! I was so patronised, I came home in a total depression. What is it about choosing to look after your own children that people consider to be such a non-event? I certainly work much harder now than I ever did – day and night (Imogen doesn't sleep much!) I don't plan to go back to work until my children are well established at school, be it primary or secondary, and I happen to believe that my son in particular really needs me. Still, it is nice to have a whinge once in a while!
Catherine, Epsom, mum to Benedict, 6 and Imogen, 2

You do seem to lose yourself when you are a full-time mum. I feel quietly embarrassed when people ask what I do, as

though my job isn't very important (and no one is interested in the fact I went to university and gave up a very good job, etc.). It is so worth it, though, especially in the winter when we can cosy up indoors and read stories.
Diane, Renfrew, mum to Aaron, 2

I had a £30,000-a-year job, commuted into London, had a mortgage and so on. In order to 'downsize', we moved into rented accommodation, and I gave up my job, took a local part-time job and haven't looked back since. I can honestly say that the drop in salary has hardly affected our household budget at all. The shocking thing is, when I did a few sums out of curiosity, the whole of my salary went on the mortgage, going out with work colleagues, sandwiches, coffee, a train season ticket and buying stupid stuff at lunchtimes just because I was out and I could. We don't want for anything – buying secondhand and seeking out bargains means that we don't have to sweat over the other stuff like money for bills, outings and toddler groups.
Victoria, Aldershot, mum to HJ, 14 months

I've been a stay-at-home mum for the last two years. When I had my eldest, I went back to work full time but after the next two children I didn't. Although financially there have been times when it has been hard (and sometimes the kids have driven me insane!), at least I have had the chance to be with them in their first few years – unlike with my eldest, where I missed out dearly with her first words and first steps as they all happened at nursery.
Frances, Halifax, mum to Sophie, 6, Emily, 2 and Jacob, 1

6 Who's Caring for Your Kids?

The vast majority of mums go back to work while our children are still small. So the chances are, at some time, we are going to have to face the Great Childcare Dilemma. We are told that if we aren't looking after our child ourselves, then it is your duty to find the best childcare possible. But what is best? Who is best? Where is best?

Lots of international research[1] attempts to show us scientifically what is best for our children, but it is hugely complex because, of course, every child is different, every

(1) Research into the effects of childcare on babies and children are reported in these two comprehensive and excellent studies:
   a) *The Effective Provision of Pre-school Education* is a five-year study of 3,000 children funded by the DfES. www.nichd.nih.gov/childcare
   (Note this in the small print: 'There was evidence that an early start in group settings, particularly before the age of two, led to slightly increased behaviour problems for a small group of children when they were three and again at five.')
   b) The National Institute of Child Health and Human Development (NICHD) published conclusions in 2006 (The NICHD Study of Early Child Care and Youth Development) having followed more than 1,000 children from birth in 1991 for fifteen years until 2006. www.nichd.nih.gov/research/supported/seccyd.cfm

childminder is different and every family is different. As yet, there are no dramatic conclusions from the researchers. But there are some key points that we need to keep at the forefront of our minds when choosing childcare.

The five golden rules for great childcare

1. Babies need lots of love, lots of one-on-one contact and lots of physical closeness.
2. Babies and toddlers need a significant other person that they can attach themselves to emotionally as a substitute when you're not there.
3. Babies and toddlers need to feel that they are very special and important to the person caring for them.
4. Your childcarer should engage in enthusiastic communication with your children – talking to them, reading to them, asking them questions, responding to their questions, challenging them to attend to others' feelings and to different ways of thinking.
5. Your child should feel calm, safe and relaxed. Studies have shown small children carrying high levels of the stress hormone cortisone in nursery settings, even though they weren't crying or looking unhappy.

All of which leads us to conclude that the *person* who will be doing the childminding is more important than the *building* in which the childcare is taking place (basic safety and hygiene aside). Remember when you gave birth? The care and attention of the midwife became everything and the decor of the maternity unit mattered little.

The childcare options

Grandparents

If you are lucky enough to have your child's grandparents living close by and they are willing to take on looking after their grandchild, there is an immediate massive advantage: no other childminder will love your child as much (apart from you). You know that your child will have the most important aspect of childcare built in from the word go – love. However, there are still some elements to be thought through and, as is so often the case, the devil is in the detail.

While your child is a little baby, the grandparent can probably cope well with the physical demands of the daily care, but what about when they are crawling? Toddling? Walking? Is the grandparent up to coping with a lively, boisterous and determined toddler, who is into everything and needs lots of exercise and stimulation?

Will the grandparent be happy to take the child to baby or toddler groups or music or gym groups? In due course, your child will need to do more than play at home with Granny. Can you find a couple of local groups, recommend them and see how that goes down? Can you suggest you go once or twice to visit these groups together? Encourage the grandparent to see it as something regular and not just an idea for 'one day'.

If the grandparent is going to care for the child in her home, you might like to look at the safety features and offer to help install them: stairgates, plug covers, cupboard locks, sharp corner covers and so on. Her house will need to be as childproofed as yours.

Grandparents have experience of bringing up children, which is wonderful, but it may also mean they have different ideas from you. Discuss with them aspects of child-rearing, such as food, sweets, discipline and routine, and make sure you agree. Perhaps they feel that a smack is OK, whereas you disagree. Or is it OK for the toddler to have a long sleep in the late afternoon so that he isn't ready for bed in the evening? As babies and toddlers and their needs change so often, perhaps you can agree to have a time every month when you sit down to discuss routines. This gives you a chance to discuss how things are going for all of you.

Are you going to pay? Perhaps you can find out the local childminders' rate and offer that, or agree a weekly fee. What are you going to do about holidays? Who chooses when holidays will be taken? Are you going to pay holiday pay? What about sickness?

Think about buggies, highchairs, car seats and other equipment. You will probably need two sets of everything – one at their house and one at yours. (You can often pick up secondhand equipment on your local Netmums Nearly New board for just a few pounds.)

Childminders

A childminder looks after a small number of children in her own home. Childminders are sometimes unfairly considered to be a form of childcare of lesser quality than expensive day nurseries. The idea of a childminder's house with a group of random children can conjure up in our minds a scene from 'The Old Woman Who Lived in a Shoe', with large groups of children swinging from rafters and swarming through the house – all completely untrue! This is a hangover from the past, when childminding was unregulated and informal.

There won't be heaps of children climbing over each other: childminders can care for only three children under the age of five at a time (and up to three more older children, but they will usually come after 'big' school). Additionally, they can have only one baby under one at any one time (although occasionally a childminder may be registered to mind two babies).

Childminders today are professional child carers. They have to be trained, formally registered, and inspected regularly by Ofsted. (It is illegal for a childminder to operate without being registered.) As well as being professional and registered, childminders are usually local mums who are also looking after their own child, or whose children are now at school.

A great advantage of childminders is that your child will be in a normal home environment. A good childminder will usually take advantage of all the local stuff to do, including toddler groups, soft play and parks. Your child also gets to play with other children, but not too many at one time.

Finding the right childminder is a little like looking for a new house: you'll get the right feeling when you've found the right childminder for you and your little one. You might see some houses that seem to tick all the right boxes, but still feel like a house and not a home. Trust your instinct.

Tips

1. Arrange to meet the childminder at her home, while the children she looks after are there.
2. Watch how she interacts with them and, more importantly, how they interact with her. Do they seem comfortable with her? Do they touch her, climb on her, sit on her lap? Do they make eye contact?
3. Ask to see her registration certificate and inspection report. Always check that the registration is up to date by asking your local Children's Information Service.
4. A good childminder will often also have a book with photos of days out, letters of reference from other mums and other things she is proud of.
5. Ask if you can speak to a mum of another child she has looked after.

6. Ask some practical questions:
   - What is the daily routine?
   - What is the weekly routine?
   - What groups and activities do they go to? Is that every week or just some weeks?
   - What do they eat?
   - Who are the other children she is looking after?
7. Ask some less practical questions too. Try to phrase them as open questions (a closed questions usually demands a yes or no answer). The aim is to get her to open up and chat so that you can learn as much as you can about her:
   - What does she do if a child won't eat lunch?
   - What would she do if a child in her care hit another child?
   - What does she do if one toddler is sleepy but they are due to go to one of their activities or groups?
   - Does she meet up with other mums at the toddler group, or other childminders? Do they come to the house?
   - What about her own children (everyone loves talking about their kids!)?

Day nurseries

Day nurseries usually offer daycare on a full-time or sessional basis, i.e. for a morning, afternoon, single day or part of the week. They may be more expensive than a childminder, but perhaps less than a nanny. Nurseries have the benefit of providing full-time daycare throughout the year – if your childminder, or her children, become sick you might find yourself without care for a while.

When looking at nurseries, bear in mind the five golden rules above (see p. 168). Don't be swayed by modern, glossy buildings with lashings of primary-coloured walls and fabulous new play equipment. Instead, ask these questions:
   - Who owns the nursery? Does the owner work in the nursery?

Alternatively, who is the manager? Has she been there long? Is it part of a chain? Ask to see the Ofsted report.

– How is the nursery structured to accommodate different age groups?

– Who are the staff caring for your child's group? Ask about each one – how old are they, what experience have they got, how long they have been at this nursery? Try to get a feel for staff turnover. A nursery with a low staff turnover is a top indication of a happy environment. It also gives some reassurance that the person your child attaches himself to will stay around for a while.

– Ask about their key worker scheme. A key worker scheme is where each child is allocated a member of staff. There are, however, different definitions of the role of a key worker. Some consider their role is to feed back to the parent on the child's progress, but this suggests the role is primarily for the parents' benefit. A real key worker should be the person whom your child bonds with, the person he trusts and identifies as his 'significant other' when you're not around, the one he goes to when he falls over or feels sad, the one who can reassure him and make him feel better. Who will this be?

– Ask if you can stay for a while and spend some time in the nursery. Watch the children and the carers interact. Get on your knees, or sit on a little chair and imagine how the nursery would look to your child. Use your instincts. Does it feel nice?

Nannies

Nannies work from your home, and they are usually qualified in childcare, or have several years' experience. Nannies may work longer hours than childminders (often 8am–6pm) and provide a continuity of care within your home that you might not get with a childminder. They can become more like one of the family and might work an occasional weekend or babysit some evenings. They are usually expected to take care of all aspects of caring for your children, including their washing, cleaning their rooms and cooking their food. You might also need to re-insure your car for the nanny to drive it, or provide petrol expenses if she has a car of her own.

There is some additional hassle (and cost) because you have to employ a nanny (they cannot be self-employed), which means you have to pay their tax. For example, if the take-home wage is £5 per hour, you need to pay her tax and National Insurance, so the gross cost ends up being about £7.50 per hour (it is usual to pay £200–£250 per week as take-home pay). You don't need to be a tax wizard though; there are companies that will manage the finances for you for £150–£200 per year. It all sounds expensive, but if you have two or more children, it can compare favourably with day nurseries. Mums working part time (or perhaps full time, and with one child) sometimes share a nanny, which makes it all more affordable.

A *daily nanny* will generally work a maximum of ten hours a day, and you might arrange for her to do some extra babysitting; she will live in her own home.

A *live-in nanny* is more likely to do babysitting as part of the job, and gives you more flexibility, but you provide her board and lodging and share your home.

It's best to agree a contract with your nanny, including the hours that she works, whether she works some time at weekends and does some babysitting. It's always good to include a list of the things she is expected to do, so everyone knows what the job entails from the start.

There is now a registration system in place for nannies, but it is voluntary and was introduced only recently. Whether or not your nanny is registered, you will need to rely on checking CVs and references thoroughly; even if you are using a nanny agency, do all the checks yourself too. Check for gaps on the CV – gaps can sometimes indicate a nanny's wish to cover up a bad job. You also could try to check out that each job listed was held by the candidate and lasted for the amount of time stated on the CV. Take up two references from other parents. If you can, speak to them as well; it might give you a better feel for the qualities of the person. Nannies should always be qualified and will usually have a BTEC qualification. Ask to see a certificate and perhaps ring their college to check that the course was completed successfully.

Try to find a number of possible nannies to interview. Make sure you look at all their qualities carefully before making a selection. If you aren't happy with any of them, keep looking at alternative options – don't just settle for the best of the bunch. Make a list of questions, like the ones below, that you want to ask each candidate. Remember to discuss what the job will involve.

1. What experience do you have?
2. How many children have you cared for and how old were they?
3. What do you find most rewarding about being a nanny?
4. What do you find most difficult about being a nanny?
5. What might a typical day be like for Jenny and John, our children?
6. What are your attitudes/practices regarding discipline and manners?
7. Are you a trained first aider?
8. What difficulties have you experienced with parents/children in live-in positions?

9. How were these resolved?
10. How many days have you had off sick in the last twelve months?
11. Do you have any experience of toilet training?
12. What is your attitude/practice as regards food/nutrition, e.g. snacks, sweets, fizzy drinks and planned, balanced meals?
13. What behaviour/developmental stages might you expect from a six to ten month old and a two year old?
14. How would you stimulate their development?
15. What would you do if:
    a. Jenny was at nursery and John was taken seriously ill?
    b. The children are playing in the garden and John requires a nappy change?
    c. Both children need a bath? How would you manage bathtime?
    d. At bathtime you find a bruise/injury on one of the children that you were not previously aware of?
    e. You found yourself getting stressed by your job?
16. Do you have any questions?

Call your best candidates (or your favoured one) back for a second interview. Give them a chance to spend some time with your children, to go through the finer details and any outstanding questions, and to get a feel for how they will work with your children.

When you have chosen your nanny, make sure you offer her the job subject to the checking of references. It's best to phone the referees (ask them if they have five minutes now or when a suitable time to call back might be). You'll learn more in five minutes on the phone than in a one-page letter. Contact other applicants and let them know that they were not successful this time.

Writing a contract can feel a bit too formal for what you want to be a nice, cosy relationship but it is really helpful to make sure that everything is agreed and understood and it stops misunderstandings before they start. Nanny agencies or nanny tax services will be able to help you with this too.

You should include:

◆ Hours of work, pay, and duties: Are you expecting your nanny to provide balanced nutritional meals for the children or to tidy away toys with the children at the end of the day?

◆ Sick pay: What happens if your nanny is off sick for two weeks? Have a clause on sick pay. For example: *'You will receive full pay for ten days in any calendar year (this will be inclusive of any statutory sick pay payable to you), thereafter only statutory sick pay will apply.'*

◆ Holiday: How are the holiday dates agreed? How far in advance? How much holiday pay do you intend to pay?

◆ Any probationary period: A three-month probationary period can be useful, as it gives you a set date when you know you can both sit down and chat about how it's going and it gives you an 'out' if it's not quite working as you'd hoped.

◆ A procedure for terminating the contract: During the probationary period, you might agree a one week's notice of termination on either side; after that four weeks' notice is usual.

Au pairs

An au pair is usually a young overseas visitor who wants to come to the country to learn the language and spend some time here. Staying with a family and helping with children and housework is a way for her to get board and lodging while she is here. An au pair will normally work about twenty-five hours a week for you. In return she will expect her own room, all meals and some pocket money – about £50 a week.

It can be lovely arrangement if you want some extra help while you are on maternity leave, some company, and a babysitter for maybe a couple of evenings a week. If you are working and have school-age children, the au pair can happily pick them up from school, play with them, give them tea and look after them until you get in from work. They are not 'cheap nannies', they are not trained in childcare and they are often very young, not much older than schoolchildren. They shouldn't be left in sole charge of young children for long periods of time. In many ways, in having an au pair you gain an extra child, albeit an older, helpful one! If you do leave young children with an au pair, make sure the au pair has someone to go to locally for support in case of difficulties and make sure they have basic first-aid training.

Most au pairs are found through agencies that match your needs with the details of the au pair. Of course, you don't get the opportunity to meet them before they arrive in the country, but you might have a chance to talk on the phone. The difficulties of checking out an individual's suitability are obvious, but it is important to do what you can to be confident in the abilities and trustworthiness of the person you are employing; ensuring the agency is reputable will help too. Go through *all the checks you can* with previous employers and with any relevant organisations, colleges and referees.

What happens next?

Discussing the care of your children can be the hardest thing in the world to do. You want it done 'your way' but as you're not actually doing it yourself, how far do you compromise? Being clear from the outset will help. Don't expect your childminder to read your mind. Say what you mean and mean what you say. If you are unhappy about something, it's important to address it early on. If you are employing a nanny, having you jointly caring for the children for the first week will help her to see how you do things, and it will give you a chance to explain your attitudes to everything from table manners to dropping litter – even things like how you stack your dishwasher and how you organise the washing can be things that will niggle for months unless you talk about them at the start!

> A useful way of keeping track of what the family is up to is to ask the childcarer to keep a daily diary, so that you can see what the children have been doing. This gives you a great start when you talk to them after work, and helps you feel part of what has been going on.

If you have a childminder, you can also start by spending a day together and then working together to settle your child over a couple of weeks. Try to build in five minutes at the start or end of each day to talk about what they've all been doing, how well he's eaten and so on.

Where to find . . .

. . . a childminder

The Children's Information Service at your local council will have a list of local registered childminders. (Phone your local council or go online to www.childcarelink.gov.uk.) They even have details of who has vacancies, but it is worth getting a complete list and calling the ones shown as full. It could be they have a place coming up very soon.

Go to your local Netmums website, where there is a Childcare board and you can see who is showing vacancies. You can put up a note yourself saying what you are looking for and asking childminders who fit the criteria to respond.

. . . a nanny

You need to decide whether to use an agency or to do the search yourself. An agency will do the legwork and find you a list of candidates, but you still need to do the interviews and check references yourself. Consider interviewing the agency first! Speak to a director and ask them for a couple of references from parents who have found a successful nanny through them.

You can find many nanny agencies on the web. Try www.nannyjob.co.uk for a list of agencies that cover your area. Alternatively, advertise in *The Lady* magazine (read by most nannies looking for work) and/or post a note (for free) on Netmums.

. . . an au pair

Contact the International Au Pair Association (IAPA) www.iapa.org or the Recruitment and Employment Confederation (REC) (www.rec.uk.com) and ask them for an agency in your area.

Police checking

Police checking is insisted upon by anyone working with children in schools and nurseries, and childminders are police-checked as part of their registration process. But if you are employing someone to work in your home as a nanny or informal carer, you should also look at having these checks done. It is quite tricky for a parent (rather than an organisation) to do this: the prospective nanny will have to complete an application, and you will need to arrange for it to be countersigned by a 'registered body'. The local council Social Services department might agree to countersign it for you. Or you can phone the Criminal Records Bureau Information Line on 0870 90 90 811 for further advice (and www.crb.gov.uk). Basically, the person is applying for a 'disclosure' from the Criminal Records

Bureau, which will contain details of relevant information held by the Police National Computer, Department of Health, Department for Education and Employment and the local police force.

Ask the Netmums:
How did you find good childcare?

The first thing to do is ask your friends for recommendations. Always go on a visit, if possible, and make sure you and your child are both made to feel welcome and you feel comfortable. Don't forget to ask to see references and don't be afraid to phone and speak to the referees. Trial and error is often the only way, as all children are different; just go with someone who makes your wee one happy.
Emma

When choosing a nursery, ask if they are happy for you to turn up any time without an appointment so you can see what really goes on. Also, if your children are already in nursery, pick them up early occasionally when they are not expecting you.
Helen, Kirklees, mum to Daniel, 5 and Lara, 3

I asked around for recommendations when I went back to work after having my first child. A friend recommended the childminder she was using for her son, so I went to visit her. I had a chat with her, checked her references and asked her a few questions about how she would care for my daughter. It was when I saw her interacting with her own kids that I just had 'mother's instinct' that she was the right childminder for my baby.
Lisa, Wolverhampton, mum to Eloise, 7 and Imogen, 5

When my son was six months, I worked part time and my sister-in-law looked after him for me for a small fee. I liked that because he wasn't going to a stranger, so I didn't feel like I was abandoning him since he was with family.
Michelle, Rochester, mum to Harry, 3 and Charlie, 16 months

It was quite a nightmare to start with but now it's fantastic. I chose childminding, as I wanted my daughter to have as normal a 'family' experience as possible. After lots of visits, I settled on the first person I visited. (I had thought she was right but needed to see the others so I had something to compare.) My daughter loves going to the house and seeing the other children. She's learning now what it's like to have a younger baby around, which I hope will help in the future too!
Sally, mum to Eve, 18 months

When I went back to work, I chose a childminder for my son. I visited nurseries but, quite frankly, I wanted him to experience real life in a home environment and to be with older children as well as younger ones. He flourished. When I was pregnant with my second child, I decided that I would stay at home but still needed to work, so I became a childminder myself. I am now three and a half years into my childminding business and enjoy every moment of having the other children here. I feel exceedingly honoured that people trust me with their most precious possessions.

At the end of the day, the choices are wide: childminders, nannies, nurseries or family. Childminders and nannies are there at all times for your children and they have a single point of contact for the time they are with them. In a nursery they will see many faces and not really know who is who, as a lot of nurseries have a huge staff turnover. A child in a nursery from baby to school time can be cared for, on average, by forty carers.

Alison, Woking, mum to Joshua, 6, Madeleine, 4 and Charlotte, 20 months

It was easy for me as I work at a nursery and that is where my son goes. I know and trust all the staff and I know it's a good nursery. I can understand how it is difficult; after all, you are trusting your child with strangers. If you're looking for childcare, I would always advise that you find a place that you feel comfortable in and where the children look happy, and that you always check out their Ofsted report first.

Kerry, Oxford, mum to Aidan, 2

7 Dirt Doesn't Matter (Much)

Do you remember how proud you were when you decorated your first home: the new Ikea sofa, the pine coffee table, the coordinated rugs and cushions, the display of candles along the mantelpiece? Your little pad never seemed to get that untidy – you were out at work all week anyway – and all it took was a couple of hours on a Saturday morning, dancing along to your favourite CD and everything was back in its perfect place and the bathroom was ready for a relaxing soak before you got ready for Saturday night.

Oh, what a contrast! The sofa and rugs now have juice stains, your candles and anything vaguely attractive have been moved from any surface that can be reached by a determined toddler. Each room is full of plastic toys of every shape and size, from toddler seesaws to chunky Lego and building bricks and a range of odd character toys from McDonald's – all of it in screaming primary colours of red, blue and yellow, which mock your carefully chosen off-white and beige decor. You can barely remember what colour the carpet is as it is permanently strewn with layers of toys, odd socks, bits of stuff from the garden and discarded clothing.

You turn your attention to one room, determined to get it in hand and sort it out once and for all. In order to tackle it, you unwisely choose to ignore the ominous silence from the rest of the house, and your one tidy room turns out to be costly: the other room has new scribbles on the walls ('It wasn't me!'), Ribena-soaked carpet and the entire contents of the toy cupboard on the floor ('I was looking for my blue train.').

As for going out anywhere, that is a trauma in itself. Only one shoe and one wellie can be found and your little one refuses to wear odd shoes (despite you suggesting what fun it would be) and so ends up in her slippers. The children's clothes cupboard seems strangely empty, although you know you've bought loads of new stuff recently – your bank statement swears you did. You rummage through the washing basket and find something less stained than the rest. You're now late, so you don't have time for make-up or hair, so you stick your hair back in a scrunchy, pull on your coat and leave the house feeling exhausted, hot and stressed before the day has even started.

Is there another way? Well, there is no way back to that calm, clean oasis that you used to call home before children (would you really want it anyway?). But there are lots of ways to make life that little bit easier. In a busy family home a little organisation goes a long way and can end up saving both time and money.

Organised mums versus disorganised mums

Many of us fall into the trap of using our home as a visual assessment of how we are coping with life as a mother. We feel we are being judged (by ourselves and others) on how neat and organised our house is. It is useful to separate motherhood from the state of the house, as this helps take the emotion and the pressure out of housework. Being disorganised and chaotic does not make you a bad mother. Being totally in control and having a perfect clean and tidy house does not make you a good mother.

Everyone is different. Maybe you are a Natural Organiser. Your home has a place for everything and everything in its place. Do you have colour-coordinated wardrobes, CD racks in alphabetical order and perfectly organised cutlery drawers?

Or are you an Inherently Untidy type? You can never find anything but can't bear to throw stuff away. Your home is probably untidy, and your life slightly chaotic. And then there is every degree in between these two types. None is better than the others; each has its strengths and weaknesses and by making just a few tweaks and adjustments, we can organise a happy family life around our natural tendencies.

It's all about finding the right balance. Highly organised mums who spend hours each day cleaning, organising, filing and colour coordinating may also find it hard to relax and sit and play with their children. You may find you need to stay in control and are stressed by normal everyday living: children's toys, even those being played with, look untidy and out of place. Children's drawings and creative art looks out of place on the walls. If this sounds like you, you probably don't need this chapter, but you might think about re-evaluating the difference between what is necessary and essential and what is unnecessary in a bid for order and control. Perhaps you can learn to let go a little. Perhaps you could redirect a little of your time and energy to getting healthily messy with your children in the park?

The rest of us could perhaps put to better use the time we spend searching for lost keys, socks, shoes and homework, and we could reduce the stress on the whole family caused by chaotic living. Being seriously disorganised, as those of us who fall into this category know only too well, is annoying, stressful and time-wasting.

Netmums' top ten organisational tips

If you do nothing else, these ten tips will make a positive difference to your home life:

1. Go with the flow. Observe where certain stuff accumulates and design the house around that rather than trying to get your family to fit your systems. For example, you may find that the children bring their drawing paper and crayons to the kitchen table and each day you have to tidy the table before tea, when you have a perfectly good children's art table in the other room. But it may be that the children want to be near you while you are cooking, or just in the same room. Can you find a place in the kitchen for a small basket or box that can be for art materials – a cupboard perhaps?

2. If space allows, have one room that is your 'good' or clean room. Have no toys in there and no food or drink at any time. Children will quickly accept this as long as you make it a general rule and never fall into the 'Well, OK, just this once' trap. There is no such thing as 'just this once'.

3. Have a nice wicker basket in every single room in the house. Use it for chucking in any toys that are on the floor of that room. Every so often you can carry a basket to the playroom or bedroom and sort through it, returning everything to its rightful home. It means that on a day-to-day basis there is always a place in every room to chuck toys when it's all getting too much or when you want to do a quick tidy up at the end of the day.

4. Have a shoe box in the hall, or porch, or utility room. Don't

even try a shoe rack – you'll spend ages putting shoes in and getting frustrated when no one else does. Have a nice basket or box (a blanket box, toy box, wicker basket or log basket) and everyone can chuck their shoes and trainers in. Also, when you're tidying up, you can throw all stray shoes in as you go.

5. Have a place for your house/car keys. Put them in the same place every single time; it will eventually become a habit and no more lost keys!

6. Never underestimate the power of flowers. If your house is getting you down, pop a bunch of fresh flowers in the room where you spend the most time. You will find your eyes drawn to them rather than the less attractive stains and scuffs.

7. Keep a bottle of washing-up liquid and a cloth in your bathroom and every day squirt and wipe round the sink and bath and shower. It takes maybe one or two minutes at most and you'll find you never have to 'clean' the bathroom.

8. Spend ten minutes on one non-essential job every day. Make it something small: clear a mantelpiece, or a small shelf, or one drawer. It is amazing how doing these jobs adds up to a clutter-free home. Don't tackle 'a room' or 'the house'. Just do this one small extra job each day. Start it and finish it.

9. Let the light in. Many of us put cleaning windows at the bottom of our long list of tasks – something to be done only if we ever get everything else done too – but it is amazing how much extra light a cleaned window lets in and the light brightens and freshens up everything in the home.

10. The housewives of the past knew a thing or two about housekeeping. Remember their wise words: 'If in doubt, throw it out' and 'If it's not beautiful or useful, get rid of it.'

Ask yourself:

What do I spend time searching for?

Make a dedicated place for that thing and always put it back in the same place. Insist the rest of the family do likewise. It is said that it takes doing something over twenty-one times before it becomes a habit but it *will* become a habit.

What causes me the most stress about household clutter and chaos?

Tackle just one thing that causes you stress and you'll have made real progress.

Ask the Netmums:

How clean is your home?

I used to vacuum, dust, clean the bathroom and iron each day. Then baby number one came along and the cleaning frenzy continued. I would vacuum with my baby in a baby sling. Then baby number two came and baby number three. The whole house was littered with toys and mess everywhere. I would vacuum at 10pm, so that it was tidy for the next day. I would also iron when they were all tucked up in bed. I was shattered!

One day it dawned on me . . . we were the only ones to notice if the house was clean and tidy, as we rarely had visitors. So what if there were toys on the floor or a bit of dust on the fire surround? What really mattered was that I wasn't shattered and spent more time with the children and less time running around the place like a headless

chicken! The cleaning frenzy stopped.
Christine, Northamptonshire, mum to Holly, 12, Chloe, 9 and Jack, 8

I must confess that I am not the most houseproud person in the world. I hoover and dust twice a week (more if we are expecting company) and I don't bother putting toys, etc., away until the children are in bed. I do washing every day and if it's dry I will put it away the same day. I very rarely do ironing (hubby does manual work so he doesn't wear dress shirts and the kids are not at school yet so they don't wear uniforms – everything else just gets folded as it dries so it doesn't get creased).
Michelle, Rochester, mum to Harry, 3 and Charlie, 16 months

As long as my kitchen stays clean and tidy, I don't care too much about the rest of the house. With an active toddler, that's about all I can hope for anyway.
Irina, Ayrshire, mum to Max, 2

I think that the most important thing is that kids can play. I'd hate to be one of those mothers that have a fit every time their child plays. I hoover every day, wash clothes and iron every day, clean the essentials daily, and cook a home-made meal every day. But the most important thing is that my kids play, make a mess and are happy.
Mary, Bristol, mum to Mollie, 4 and Connie, 19 months

I meet myself coming back! I vacuum at least once a day, the washing machine is on all day and the dishwasher is on all the time. There are only three of us, but I seem to be cleaning and tidying all the time. I know I should leave it and spend more time with my little one, but if I see things need cleaning I have to do it. My house never looks tidy though!

Caroline, Wakefield, mum to James, 3

I concentrate on my kitchen and living room on a daily basis. I like to get my washing-up done and clean down my work surfaces. I hoover every day and straighten up generally in the living room because that's where we relax in the evenings. The upstairs is a different matter. On a daily basis I make the beds but don't pay too much attention to upstairs during the week! I do the bathroom thoroughly once a week but put bleach down the loos every couple of days.

Michelle, Hertfordshire, mum to Carly, 8 and Paige, 4

Life's too short to clean. The kitchen floor gets mopped when my daughter says, 'This floor is sticky', and the hoover comes out when the cats have had a fight and there's fur everywhere. I tidy her toys up in the evening but that's only because she likes to wreck everywhere all over again the next day. She often asks me for a cloth and sets off dusting. Do you think she's trying to tell me something?

Helen, Congleton, mum to Willow, 3

I've never really been very good at finding the inclination to do the cleaning/tidying, but since having my son, I've realised that it would be very lazy and selfish of me to bring him up in a messy, dirty house. I have a four-week cleaning rota that includes all the daily, two-day, weekly and monthly tasks, and I make sure they're all done

before I go to bed! I've noticed a real difference in the appearance of my house. I don't think, 'It can wait till tomorrow', as that never happens with me!
Amy, Grantham, mum to Cameron, 17 months

I can never find time to do cleaning. I always used to hoover every day, dust every other day, clean the bathroom and upstairs once a week and do the ironing once a week when Cameron would have a nap during the day. Now I haven't hoovered for three days, haven't dusted for about four and I'm very ashamed to say I haven't cleaned the bathroom, cleaned upstairs or done any ironing for about two weeks. I just can't find the time to do anything. I work till 6pm four days a week and most weekends and when I come home I just want to spend some time with Cameron before he goes to bed. We very rarely get any visitors and most things are left for me to do around the house. My other half does the dishes and that's about as far as his cleaning goes. He will clean up the kitchen if it's quite bad, but I'm fed up with everything being left for me to do all the time, so it just doesn't get done! I've got a day off tomorrow though, so I will attempt to give the place a good cleaning.
Rhia, Neath, mum to Cameron, 2

I do the kitchen and lounge every day. I wash up after every meal, wipe the surfaces, hoover the kitchen and lounge, and dust the lounge. Every Monday, Wednesday and Friday I mop the kitchen and lounge floors. Then I choose one room upstairs to do a day; I have our room, Mark's room and the bathroom. The spare room I can't get into yet, but when we sort it for the new baby then I will squeeze that one in too. Sometimes I feel lazy during the day so I don't do it until Mark is in bed. Mark helps; if he sees me tidying up, he will put his toys away for me, so doing his room is easy – I just hoover and dust. If I have an energy spurt, then I do the whole house – even sweep the garden.

Claire, Shaftesbury, mum to Mark, 22 months

The cleaning will still be there when they are three and in school! Just make sure that you have clean clothes and food in the fridge. Anything else is a bonus. (I was going to add clean dishes to eat off, but I've discovered picnics, both out and about and on a blanket on the living-room floor – much more exciting!)

Bethan, Swansea, mum to Abigail, 2 and Oliver, 1

We have a cleaning rota in our house. It got to the point where I was sooooo sick of things not being done to my standard that I split the house into zones (à la FlyLady, www.flylady.net) and wrote what needed to be done per zone. Then every day we do a zone each after brekkie and Maia is chief duster. It sounds sad, I know, but it keeps me sane.

Tracy, Wolverhampton, mum to Maia, 2, and Cadence 4 weeks

My top tip is not to leave a room empty-handed, and it works, because I find when my house is tidy, it's easier to keep it that way. I also now set myself a time limit for each room, as it used to take me all day to clean, and sometimes the evening too! When I know I've got only an hour to do the living room, for example, I do manage to finish in that time.

Tina, Kent, mum to Saffron, 20, Simon, 18, Daisy, 2 and full-time stepchildren Jessica, 10 and Fleur, 9

'Cleaning the house while kids are still growing
Is like shovelling snow when it is still snowing.'
So I don't bother!
Jodie, Milton Keynes, mum to Adam, 9 and Samuel, 3

I clean my kitchen every day for hygiene reasons; my front room gets hoovered every day; the rest of the house is a tip! Do I care? No! Are my kids happy? Yes! And that's all that matters!
Sarah, Colchester, mum to Megan, 4 and Poppy, 15 months

My routines are all from FlyLady (www.flylady.net) and I can't speak highly enough of her! I used to loathe any form of housework and resented every second I spent doing it. As a result, my house used to get really untidy and every week I spent a whole day making myself miserable by forcing myself to do the entire week's worth in one go. Now, however . . .

I make sure I do at least one load of laundry a day – that means washed, dried, folded and either put away or added to the Ironing Mountain I keep in my husband's study (out of sight and I refuse to feel guilty – I iron maybe twice a week, when my husband runs out of shirts or whenever the mood takes me). I often put the washing in the night before and set the timer so that it finishes just as I'm getting up; that way I can hang it out first thing and forget about it until later (or until it rains). I usually load the bread maker at the same time and put that on timer too, so we can wake up to fresh bread – yummy!

I sweep the kitchen floor every morning and mop once a week unless it needs doing sooner. I routinely dust and vacuum once a week unless it needs doing in between.

When I do my weekly dusting and vacuuming, I spend ten minutes downstairs and ten minutes upstairs – tops. Then every now and again I give each room a really thorough going over.

But the best routine I've ever started is the morning 'swish and swipe' in the bathroom . . . Once I'm done getting showered and cleaning teeth, etc., I run the loo brush around the bowl and use damp loo roll to wipe the seat and around the rim. Then I wipe down the sink and taps with the towel I've used before I throw it in the wash. I wipe round the bath in the evening during bathtime and give the shower a quick buff in the morning while I'm in there. I can't remember the last time I actually 'cleaned the bathroom' and it's always sparkly.

If I ever don't feel like doing tidying or cleaning or anything unpleasant, I just make myself do five minutes and then stop and do something nice for the next ten minutes. Then I do another five and then fun again for ten . . . it's amazing how much you can do without really feeling like you are doing anything.

Dawn, Halifax, mum to Sam, 12 and Alex 10 months

I get stressed if I can't keep the house tidy and I can't sit still if I know there are dishes in the sink. But developing Obsessive Compulsive Disorder after child number one is what started it all off – before that I didn't own a duster!

Joanna, Bristol, mum to Alannah, 10 and Johnny, 7

I have to admit to being a bit of a slob when it comes to housework. Yes, the state of the house bothers me but I don't see why I should always do it. When I was pregnant, my husband announced that he thought it was great because I would have to keep the house clean once we had a baby, and I did for a while. The most I did was one week beyond my due date when I cleaned out all the cupboards and baked lots of cakes! Now my son is two and I can't keep up.

I work from home, which doesn't help, as every spare minute is spent keeping my business going. I do have an excuse: my son is scared of the vacuum cleaner, so we can do that only when he isn't around. My top tip for getting yourself to do the housework is to invite friends/mothers, etc. around regularly. I belong to the National Childbirth Trust and at least once a month I host coffee at my house. As several people are allergic to my cats, it means I have to vacuum and dust everywhere (downstairs) before they arrive – so it does get done periodically!
Claire, Worksop, mum to Luke, 2

I like my kitchen, living room and downstairs toilet to be clean and tidy; these are the only areas visitors see anyway. I'm not too fussed about upstairs as long as the bathroom is clean. I think as long as my kitchen is clean and the toilet (I'd hate to be like the advert about the smelly toilet!), then I'm happy. I'd rather spend time with my daughter.
Susan, Dudley, mum to Emma, 1

I have started to chill out about housework now. When I had my first baby, the house was really clean. Now I've had my fourth, I just don't find the time and think there are more important things in life than cleaning – like having fun with the kids. And when I do clean up, the kids only mess it up again!
Lisa, St Neots, mum to Andrew, 12, Emma, 9, Matthew, 7 and Adam, 2

Ask yourself:

Often we are overwhelmed by how much there is to do and we wait until we get a clear stretch of time to have a complete spring clean. It's so much better to do a little each day, and that way you will find you are keeping on top of things with very little extra effort.

Can you sit down and have a think about tasks and duties in the home? Divide these into three areas: essential, useful and life's too short? Keep this list beside the kettle for a few days and add to it as you go along – you won't think of everything straight away. For each job you do, allocate it to one of the three categories. For each job you notice needs to be done but you don't get to do, put it in a category.

This system might help:

Essential
For example:
– Feeding the kids
– Having clean underwear for the whole family
– Getting to school on time

Useful
For example:
– Cleaning the fridge
– Washing the kitchen floor
– Cleaning out the broom cupboard/under the stairs
– Sorting the linen cupboard

Life's too short
For example:
– Home-made pasta
– Darning socks

When you think the list is complete, sit down with a coffee and review it. Move things from one category to another if appropriate. Can you commit to keeping up to date with the Essential list each day/week? Can you spend just *fifteen minutes each day* on the Useful list? Go through it item by item, doing one thing each day.

A happy, healthy house

In looking at how to be a happy mum and a happy family, we should give just a little attention to our home. If our home was a living thing, what would make it happy? Of course, it isn't truly alive, but perhaps we can introduce some positive energy. At the very least we can make it a healthy, clean environment for us and our children.

As well as being tested on animals (bad karma), many cleaners contain a cocktail of chemicals, which can irritate your skin and also destroy friendly as well as dangerous germs. There are growing concerns as to the effect these chemicals have on eczema and asthma as well as skin allergies. You can safely involve your children in cleaning using the tips, ingredients and ideas below and it is a perfect introduction to showing your children how easy it is to work with the planet with not a flowery skirt in sight!

Baking soda (bicarbonate of soda)

This breaks down grease and is great added to vinegar or lemon juice to make them more abrasive. It is also a great deodoriser in fridges and dishwashers as well as a water softener.

- Mix it with a bit of water to dissolve grease and grime.
- Use it dry on carpets to lift out stains.
- You can neutralise most strong odours with it.
- Use it on a damp sponge to remove stains on general surfaces.
- For blocked drains, sprinkle some over the plug holes and then pour in some vinegar.
- It can also be sprinkled on carpets before vacuuming to freshen them up.

Olive oil

Use olive oil to get rid of finger marks on stainless steel surfaces and utensils. Put some on a kitchen towel and rub it over the finger marks.

White vinegar (or, better still, white wine vinegar)

Think of this as your all-purpose cleaner. It will clean and deodorise as it goes.

- Use 50/50 mixed with water as a cleaner in your bathroom and kitchen.
- Put an eggcup full in your washing machine instead of softener.
- It's great for towels or cloth nappies, as the coating a fabric softener gives them makes them less absorbent.
- It's a great descaler. Soak paper towels in the vinegar, wrap them around taps, cover with plastic bags and secure with an elastic band and leave them there for a few hours – the taps will come out looking brand new.

Lemon juice

Use this to dissolve scum, particularly in hard-water areas. It can be mixed with vinegar and/or bicarbonate of soda to make a cleaning liquid that will get rid of serious stains and is also useful as a bleaching agent.

◆ Mix one cup of olive oil with half a cup of lemon juice and pour it into a spray bottle to use as furniture polish. Spray a little on the surface and then rub it all over. The lemon juice cuts through the dirt and the olive oil gives a nice shine. Buff with a dry cloth.

◆ Lemon juice is also good for microwave smells: add a few slices of lemon to a bowl of water and microwave on high power for a couple of minutes.

Essential oils

◆ If you soak nappies, try a couple of drops of tea tree oil instead of bleach. It will make them last a lot longer.

◆ Throw out your antibacterial spray and create your own using a couple of drops of lavender, a couple of drops of tea tree and some eucalyptus oil in the winter or citronella in the summer (to deter flies).

◆ Put a few drops of essential oil into home-made playdough to make it smell nice – lavender perhaps, or eucalyptus in the wintertime to help fight colds.

More tips

◆ Light a candle to help get rid of smells (be careful with children and naked flames).

◆ Consider using eco-balls instead of washing powder or liquid in your machine. These are great if your child has sensitive skin.

◆ When you replace your white goods, buy the most economical one you can – 'A' being best.

◆ Use the washing line when you can, but when you must use the tumble dryer try using dryer balls. They shorten drying time and soften fabric.

- Clean your windows with vinegar and water.
- A steam cleaner can be a great way of cleaning without chemicals.
- Sunlight can be used to bleach out stains.

Staying on top

Laundry

Decide how often you ought to be putting a wash on in order to stay on top of the washing: every day, every second day, twice a day? Whatever it is, put that under your essential items. Realising that you need to do a wash every day is a good start. If you miss one, you need to do two the next time so you don't fall behind and end up overwhelmed by a mountain of washing.

Tips
- Don't overload the washing machine: it makes everything more creased.
- Don't tumble dry unless you have to – it's expensive, for a start, and it's harder on your clothes than letting them air dry. The clothes will also collect much more static electricity.
- Give clothes a good shake to remove creases and fold out any remaining creases with your hands as you hang them out.
- Fold sheets to the size of half a pillowcase before you put them in the washing machine. They'll come out hardly creased.

Ironing

Unless you find it therapeutic (yes, we have met mums who like ironing!) then keep ironing to an absolute minimum. Obviously, smart work shirts need ironing but most children's clothes do not; neither do pyjamas, sheets, jeans, most T-shirts or knitwear. Wash and dry them properly, fold them and put them away.

If you and your partner both need your work clothes ironed,

consider a local ironing service. Most are run by local mums looking to earn an extra few pounds and the service is relatively inexpensive – maybe £14 for twenty shirts or thereabouts. Calling in this service even once every three or four weeks can be a huge help.

Odd socks

Odd socks have driven many a mum to madness! We all agree we have a black hole that sucks in odd socks and we publicly admit that we accept defeat. This is a problem that can never be eliminated, but it can be reduced.

Tips
- Train everyone in the house to put their socks together as they take them off and before they go in the wash basket.
- Don't put any sock into the washing machine that doesn't have a partner; that way, no odd socks should come out (in theory!).
- Colour-code socks. For example, your partner has all black socks of the same type, so you can match any Daddy-sock to any other Daddy-sock. If you have more than one child, give each one a base colour – blue or pink, for example – and only buy socks in that colour for that child. This way you eliminate the time-wasting 'Whose sock is whose?' activity.
- Have an odd-sock bag and get it out regularly, pour it on the kitchen table and get the children to help with the aid of chocolate buttons – for each pair found the child gets a chocolate button.

Putting clothing away

This really is a task that is best done every day, but do it only once a day. Otherwise, you could follow your children around, picking up cardigans and discarded items and putting them away all day!

Put freshly washed clothes on a bed or on the landing; next to it add a pile of clothes that you've picked up around the house and bathroom. Tackle the whole lot at the same time – perhaps while the children are in the bath, if they are old enough to be left on their own, or just afterwards when they are relaxed and can play quietly in their room while you potter around them. If clothes have been worn but aren't dirty, fold them and put them away: it's good for the environment and reduces the amount of laundry. It helps to remember that in 'the old days' it was common for children to have just one or two outfits for the week and a change for Sundays.

Paperwork
Tips
- Deal with school letters, forms, permission slips, requests for money, school trips, etc. as soon as they come in, i.e. that very afternoon, and send them back to school the next day whenever possible.
- Have an in-tray: put bills that need to be paid, calls that need to be made, insurance that needs to be sorted, queries and so on in it.
- Set aside a little time twice a week to deal with paperwork.
- The business desk rule of 'don't touch a piece of paper more than once' is good for home paperwork too. Avoid the 'I'll just put it here for now' trap. When you sit down with your in-tray, no piece of paper should be returned to the tray. It should be dealt with, filed or thrown away.
- Have a supply of stamps, envelopes and writing paper in the same place as your chequebook.
- Get as many bills and outgoings as possible put on direct debit.
- Put all receipts into an envelope and sort through them every month or few months.
- Have a filing system – one place for all your paperwork with

subdivisions. This can be a cardboard box and some cardboard A4 folders: one for cars (tax, insurance, MOT, log books, etc.); one for tax (P45s, P60s, tax forms, letters, etc.); and one for utility bills (gas, electricity, phone, etc.).

Appointments

A family calendar is not just useful, it's essential. Missing an occasional doctor's or dentist's appointment is just about forgivable but missing a friend's child's birthday party or your own child's school play or sports day is something you can't risk.

Tips
– Have your family calendar or wall planner in a very prominent position – probably in the kitchen, near where you have breakfast.
– Have a pen attached to it, even if it is a DIY job with a bit of string and a drawing pin.
– Write appointments in straight away and train yourself to look at it every day – morning and evening!
– If you don't trust yourself, most mobile phones can be programmed to send you a text on a certain date, i.e. the day before a birthday, deadline or event.

Children's parties

The first year or so, being invited to a children's party is a novelty and we enjoy choosing the perfect gift, wrapping it in colour co-ordinated wrapping paper and including a personalised card. But with the current fashion being to invite the whole class, that's potentially thirty parties per child! If you add in a selection of relatives and outside-of-school friends, a mum of two could well be dealing with a hundred parties and presents a year! So a little planning and organisation is not just nice but really essential.

Tips
- Put your friends' children's birthdays on your planner.
- Buy cards in bulk: you can buy a box of mixed birthday cards and keep it topped up so you've always got a boy or girl card to hand.
- When you have an art session with the children, make cards and put them away. Home-made cards mean so much to grand-parents, aunts, etc.
- Also buy wrapping paper in bulk – keep a few rolls in stock.
- Start a present drawer. When you're out and see something suitable, maybe on special offer, buy one or even more depending on your cash flow, and keep them in your present drawer. After Christmas, there are always great bargains on leftover stocking fillers and all year round the supermarkets have an aisle of cheap toys.

Four really useful things

Collect and collate the contents of these:

1. A VIP (Very Important Paperwork) box
Have a special place designated for passports, birth certificates, driving licences, chequebooks, paying-in books, savings books . . .

2. A first-aid kit
An old biscuit box makes a great first-aid box. Gather the essentials: antibacterial cream (with local anaesthetic), insect sting cream, plasters, thermometer, bottle of Rescue Remedy, arnica cream for bruises, cotton wool for cleaning cuts.

3. A list of phone numbers
You need your list of phone numbers in an easily accessible place where it isn't going to get lost. If your child is at school, bring a

piece of paper and pen and jot down as many mums' phone numbers and mobile numbers as possible. Record RSVP numbers from party invitations. If you have them in your mobile, that's fine, but if you lose your phone you've lost lots of important data. A top tip is to start an Excel spreadsheet on your computer and add all your names and numbers to it as well as to your mobile. Update it as often as you get a new number. You can also print a copy off for the wall or the fridge.

4. Mum's box of useful stuff

Put the following items on your shopping list and assemble them over the next few weeks. Think about what else you might find useful. Put everything in a box or a drawer or even a bag hung in a cupboard under the stairs – ideally in a secret location! If your partner already has these things, you might want to get your own as well; it's often when the household one goes missing that your secret box really comes into its own.

– Safety pins
– A sewing kit (with multi-coloured threads) – even one out of a Christmas cracker
– Screwdrivers. Either pick up a cheap multi-purpose screwdriver in the DIY shop (the ones with different heads are good) or even those mini-packs that you get (again) in crackers can come in handy
– Tweezers
– A torch
– Spare batteries (a selection of sizes, including the ever-useful AAA, AA)
– Some candles
– Boxes of matches
– A spare set of keys
– A tape measure

– Scissors
– Tape
– A corkscrew!

Food and shopping

Do you regularly open the fridge hoping for inspiration for this evening's dinner only to find it looking like Old Mother Hubbard's cupboard? Do you wander aimlessly round the supermarket, or stare blankly at an incomplete shopping list? A family meal planner could revolutionise your life (well, the teatime bit of it at least!). It takes a little bit of effort. You'll need to find half an hour to think 'food thoughts', but many of our mums have declared this a resounding success.

	Week 1	Week 2	Week 3	Week 4
Monday				
Tuesday				
Wednesday				
Thursday				
Friday				

- ◆ Each week includes only five planned days. Weekends are left free so you can go to the shop and choose something you fancy or get a takeaway, or eat with friends.
- ◆ On a rough piece of paper, list twenty meals that your family enjoys. Do it in groups of four or five food types, so starting with pasta, find four pasta dishes for your list, then maybe chicken dishes, then fish. Simple foods like pizza or sausages can be listed as well as more substantial meals like roasts.
- ◆ Now, take your chart and start to fill in the boxes from your list.

Roughly balance the weeks by including a pasta dish, a chicken recipe, a veggie dish and a fish recipe each week.

◆ Add matching accompaniments to each dish, such as potatoes – boiled, baked, roast or chipped. And balance the meal with a vegetable and a pudding.

◆ You can now write next week's shopping list from the first week of your planner.

The school morning

Here are some tips to help, both with starting school for the first time and with managing school mornings. Do all this the night before and mornings will be much less frantic:

– Choose and lay out your own clothes for the next day (including tights, bra, etc.)

– Choose and lay out your child's or children's clothes, including any hairbands.

– Prepare any packed lunches.

– Check the calendar for the next day and see if anything extra is needed, such as swimming stuff.

– Check shoes are in place.

– Have school bags or children's bags ready with their homework, any forms that need to be returned, favourite toy or possessions for little ones.

And on the day . . .

◆ Ask your children to put their clothes or uniform on before coming down for breakfast – it will save a lot of time.

◆ Many parents don't let their children watch television until they are completely ready to go (including coat!). Write down all that this includes: getting dressed, eating breakfast, doing teeth, brushing hair, washing face, making bed, putting shoes on, checking bags.

◆ As something different once in a while, you could make a little checklist for them to carry around – they love ticking things off as they do them. Or use a star chart for a couple of weeks to help get them into the routine; or an occasional sticker to wear on their coat could be a reward when you've had a good morning. (Remember to give yourself a pat on the back too!)

◆ Have fun too. Try to intercept a tricky day: could you make up a game where they put all their white clothes on first, followed by grey? Or put on a song and set them a challenge to dance while getting dressed at the same time – they have to have at least four items of clothing on for each song played.

◆ Make some things into a race (it might be best if they race against you, rather than against each other). Say, 'I bet I can tidy up the breakfast things before you've put your shoes on', or 'Can you put your cardigan on before I count to ten?'

◆ Keeping a packet of wipes, a hairbrush, toothbrushes and children's toothpaste in the kitchen can save a last dash upstairs.

◆ If your children need help with getting dressed and ready, do one person at a time, including yourself, from start to finish rather than doing a bit of everybody. It saves time in the long run.

Make your home school-friendly

Once your children are at school the amount of paperwork and additional kit and caboodle increases dramatically. Here are some tips for keeping it under control:

1. Get a white board (or a piece of paper) and write down the weekly timetable of all your children's activities. Put it on the wall so that you can see at a glance what you need each day.

2. Create a folder for notes from school, newsletters, forms, etc.

Make sure any forms that need action are at the front of the folder.

3. Make a space for book bags.
4. Designate a filing tray or folder for homework – one for each child if necessary. Keep the school folder in one of these.
5. Make sure you have enough envelopes to return school notes for the whole year. It sounds silly, but it's so irritating when you're in a hurry and you've run out.
6. Have a box for the uniform at the end of each child's bed. It makes finding everything much easier.
7. As soon as children get home from school on Friday, put the uniform in the wash. Iron it on Saturday if you have to iron it at all, so it is ready to be put out on Sunday night.

A final thought

When the house and all it involves is really driving you mad, take time out to ask yourself: what is really going on here? Frantic tidying, cleaning and feeling anxious about the state of the house are classic signs of stress –an attempt to get back on top of things when you are feeling like control of your life is slipping. Your actions could be an attempt to claw back emotional control by focusing on your immediate physical environment. If this is the case, no amount of cleaning will bring you the peace of mind you are craving. You'll just end up exhausted.

Ask yourself:

Are you OK?

When you find yourself getting stressed about the house, can you sit down for a moment? Breathe deeply and ask yourself: 'What am I feeling? How am I feeling? What is really going on

with me? What is on my mind? What am I worried about?'
What would help you to feel better about that situation? Is
there someone you can talk to about it? Read Chapter 9,
Beating the Blues.

If you get a day when the house is in complete chaos, the walls are
closing in and it's all making you feel like screaming – stop and do
something completely different. Pack a picnic, and if it's a nice day,
go to the park, or if it's raining put your wellies on and go and
splash in puddles and picnic in the car. Or phone a friend and tell
her you can't stay indoors another moment and invite yourself
round for coffee. You're not going to achieve anything useful in this
mood, so the general consensus is the best thing to do is just get
out of the house. Yes, it'll all still be there when you get back, but
if you've had a chat or a laugh, had some fresh air or looked up at
the sky, you will find your sense of perspective has been restored
and you can see it for what it is: household chores that just don't
matter (much).

8 What About Me?

In recent Netmums' research[1], lack of me-time was shown to be the number one stress factor for 75 per cent of mums. More than lack of sleep, or any other of the more obvious stressors, lack of me-time wins the Enemy Number One slot.

It's not surprising really. It seems we go almost overnight from being young, free and single with time for long baths, clothes shopping, leisurely dinners in restaurants, Sunday lunchtime in the pub and weekend lie-ins (sigh) to being on call and on duty twenty-four hours a day seven days a week – no evenings off, no weekends off, not even bank holidays off. We have these tiny little people for whom we are totally responsible, who see us as the centre of their universe, who want to be with us every minute of the day and who demand our attention every second. It's our job to make sure they are emotionally secure, physically healthy and well and to cover all the daily basics of feeding, washing and clothing. Even if the children aren't with us, they are on our minds – we even sleep

(1) Netmums' research, *A Mum's Life*, published 2004

with one ear open. And we have a home that needs to be kept clean, laundry that needs to be washed and ironed and put away, food that needs to be bought, prepared and cooked, children that need to be played with, homework that needs to be supervised, and, very likely, a paid job to fit in somewhere too.

Before going any further, we have to face up to something. It's the intrinsic, basic nature of a mum to put herself last – and even reading and thinking about me-time probably gives you a little stab of guilt and a feeling that it isn't quite appropriate for you to be reading this. That little voice is whispering to you that:

◆ Me-time is selfish time. Good mums don't do that.
◆ You're so lucky to have such lovely children, how could you need time off?
◆ There are much more urgent things to be done.
◆ I can't afford to relax, I've got to stay on top of everything – who else is going to do it?
◆ Being a good mum means looking after everyone else first.
◆ Me-time would be nice but it's not feasible at the moment.

Ask yourself:

Is the problem more than a lack of me-time?

It might be helpful for you to consider what happens to you when you've had no time for yourself. Do you feel . . .

Resentful	On edge
Exhausted	Snappy
Irritable	Agitated
Angry	Stressed
Bitter	Discontented
Trapped	Unfulfilled?

How many of these emotions do you regularly feel rising up within you? It may be that they are deep down inside, but you push them away and instead engage in yet more frenetic activity in an effort to get on top of things. You think that when you get a bit more organised, you'll be able to loosen up a bit and take some time out . . . but no matter how much you do, you never seem to get to the bottom of the pile. And so you feel even more tired and even more resentful. You snap at the children and then you feel guilty. So you try a bit harder . . . STOP!

If you regularly feel any one or more of these emotions, take it as a red flag that you are doing too much. Ask yourself every day: 'What have I done for myself today?'

Have you ever wondered why, on an airplane, we are advised that in the event of an emergency, mothers should put the oxygen mask on themselves first, before their children? There is a need to take care of and cherish ourselves in order to be able to nurture and cherish our children.

Taking care of yourself doesn't mean you stop loving your children, or that you are a bad wife or mother. In fact, it will make you an even better one.

You will have more energy, more laughter, more joy to share with them. And you are showing your children, by example, that it is OK for mums to take time for themselves, that it is good to value yourself. Good mums don't have to be martyrs to motherhood, sacrificing their own lives in the process. You are your children's role model. Your little girl will learn that one day when she becomes a mum, she doesn't have to choose between being a good mum or a happy mum, and she will be better equipped to look after herself as well as her future family as a result, and your little boy will have greater respect for and realistic expectations of his future partner.

Making time for you: the difference between urgent and important

If you own a car, think of all the care that goes into keeping it roadworthy. You regularly have to fill it up with petrol, and check and maintain the battery, windscreen washers and tyre pressures. You even wash it so it looks nice. You don't drive it too hard or rev it too much. You take decent care of it knowing that that is how to get the best out of it. We consider that giving our car a decent level of time, money and care is necessary and important. And yet how much more important are you than a car! How much more important is it that you are fit and well and 'roadworthy'?

Although it doesn't seem *urgent* to spend some time on yourself, it is really *important*. It is really important that you redress your time deficit and start to take care of yourself. Otherwise, your health, both emotionally and physically, will suffer and it will become urgent – like a broken-down car.

So, where do you start with this business of looking after yourself?

The first change you need to make is a change of *mindset*. It means accepting that you do need to take care of yourself. It means making a commitment to do this. It means putting time for you on the list along with the other jobs that have to be done each day: washing up, cooking tea, making the beds, me-time. Once you've made that commitment to yourself, the next step is figuring out when and how. Find a time of day that suits you and your family, then it is more likely that it will happen. If you have a regular time slot, you will be able to plan for it and look forward to it. It will be a time to do whatever you would like or need to do for yourself, and it will probably become known as 'Mum's Time'.

If, for some reason, your time looks like it is not going to happen, negotiate another time slot with yourself and/or your partner straight away so that it becomes the norm that you need time for yourself, just as much as you need the air that you breathe and the food that you eat. It might take the rest of the family a little while to get used to it, especially if you've spent months or years putting yourself at the back of the queue. Tell yourself you are doing this for them as well as for yourself.

Ask yourself:

Has it been a good day?

Spend a few minutes at the end of each day writing down three things you've done that day that make you a good mum. Try to be specific and focus on the little things that you did that seem insignificant but are actually important. Did you make a healthy tea when a frozen pizza would have been easier? Did you take them to the park when you'd rather have sat and watched TV? Did you make them laugh by playing with the bubbles at bathtime? Did you use imagination and humour to get them into their car seats when you really wanted to shout?

Keep this list by your bed and try to make a new list every day for at least seven days or longer if you can. Reading back over a week's worth of entries should give you the reassurance you need that you are doing a great job and that you deserve a little time for yourself.

Ask the Netmums:
How do you find some me-time?

After years of no me-time, I decided I had to have some time to myself to save my sanity! I joined a jewellery-making evening class at my local adult education centre, which is something I had always wanted to do, but never got round to. On my 'night off' my husband puts the kids to bed and I go out and get creative! I have met some lovely people on the course (not just mums with young kids!) and get a real sense of achievement out of designing and making my own jewellery.
Lisa, Wolverhampton, mum to Eloise, 7 and Imogen, 5

I'm really lucky, as my partner is around a fair bit and helps with the little ones a lot. We tend to split bedtimes between us, each of us responsible for one child, and most evenings we manage to have them down by 7.30, so after we've cleared up I have the evening for us/me. I do know, though, that not everyone has this help and support. As I said, I'm really lucky. I think it's a case of grabbing me-time as and when you can. I have a lovely twenty minutes in the morning; when the boys eat their brekkie, I sit with a cuppa and yesterday's paper!
Jenny, Canterbury, mum to Benjamin, 3 and James, 18 months

I'm a single mum, so me-time is spent after my daughter is tucked up in bed – sometimes it even includes a Bacardi and Coke, a long soak in the bath or a takeaway. When she was small, I did an online computer course, which gave me some other focus; now I spend the time on Netmums! I try to do the clearing up and tidying before she goes to bed, then I turn my back on any mess and relax in front of the TV and computer.

Louise, North Staffordshire, mum to Grace, 3

I am a stay-at-home mum and my other half works five days a week. I've managed to agree three hours Saturday mornings and three hours Sunday afternoons me-time. I have just enrolled on a Learn Direct course and have arranged to see my tutor once a week (on Saturday morning). I noticed straight away how quiet and calm it all was – a child-free environment . . . ahh, bliss! Also, when the children are in bed, it is nice to curl up with a bottle of wine and some chocolate.

Sam, Wolverhampton, mum to Alex, 9, Hollie, 7 and Lewis, 4

I'm lucky now that the children are all at school, as in theory from 9am to 3pm is me-time. But, as all stay-at-home mums know, there is always so much to do: washing, ironing, shopping for food (boring!) and lots of other chores. By the time the kids get home I'm usually tired out. I've never had what I'd call proper me-time, like a hairdresser's appointment or facial, or been able to do a course . . . so sad! My me-time is when the kids are asleep in bed (usually by 8.30pm). Then I crash out on the sofa with a glass of wine and a bar of chocolate, which is my little treat.

Christine, Northamptonshire, mum to Holly, 12, Chloe, 9 and Jack, 8

I'm only just getting me-time after spending the last seven years bringing my children up on my own. I had four children under five and was on my own from day one, so never got a minute. They had a good bedtime routine, but once they were asleep it was housework, washing, ironing, etc. My youngest two are now at nursery, so I get five sessions of me-time a week. I can finally go to the toilet on my own! But I have forgotten how to be 'me', as I'm so used to being 'mum'. I miss the children dreadfully, and feel really lonely when they are not with me. I am hoping I will get used to it, and be able to find myself again.

Laura, Folkestone, mum to Courtney, 7, Reece, 6 and twins Jayden and Chloe, 3

When Sam was first born and I was breastfeeding what felt like constantly, me-time was scarce and finding some was a necessity to keep me sane. What I used to do at the end of the day was get in the bath with Sam and breastfeed him in there, then my husband would come and take him from me and put him to bed while I topped up the bath and soaked for hours at a time with a book. I can still remember the feeling a few weeks into motherhood of being able to relax and read again; it felt great, like I'd really achieved something!

When Sam was older and Emma came along, I took to going out one afternoon at the weekend just for a couple of hours to wander round town. I made sure I always bought myself something, even if it was just a cheap lipstick or a pair of earrings from the market. I also loved having a coffee in a café with no kids in sight and being able to read a magazine in peace.

Donna, Rotherham, mum to Samuel, 5 and Emma, 3

After my second son was born, I had post-natal depression. My health visitor suggested, as I already used the services of a childminder for two afternoons a week while I went to work, that I extend one of the afternoons to a full day, so in the morning I could do whatever I wanted, i.e. go to town, do nothing or go to the gym, then go to work in the afternoon. I know it cost me extra but it was well worth it.
Susan, Derby, mum to Jack, 8 and Nathan, 3

I get me-time on a Monday evening when I go to Keep Fit with friends. It's a couple of hours for me to chat to friends about adult things with a bit of exercise thrown in.
Michelle, Rochester, mum to Harry, 3 and Charlie, 16 months

Even with my mum living next door and helping out, I still needed a whole day with the baby in nursery. I thought it was going to be time for catching up with housework but quickly realised that I needed some time to do nothing. Only when I started to have that time – having a nap or going out for lunch with a friend – did I completely recover from having post-natal depression. I also book my little sweetie into a crèche while I do aerobics once per week. I find that exercise is essential for my happiness and well-being!
Kerry, Halifax, mum to Oliver, 5 and Daisy, 17 months

I think it's really important to have me-time. It's so easy to forget that you're you still and not just 'mum'! I work a couple of days a week, so that gets me out and about, and my mum and dad have the little man once a month so me and hubby can either go out together or separately – can't beat a girly night out! I just started Slimming World last week, so that'll be an evening out doing something for myself, as

well as getting slimmer (hopefully!). Oh, and I go to bingo
every other week, so I don't do too badly, do I?
Wendy, Castleford, mum to Edward, 3

I remember when my two were very little – six months and
two and a half. I had to have over an hour's worth of root
canal treatment and I was actually looking forward to it
'cos it meant some time off!
Rachel, Poole, mum to Alix, 7 and Eliiott, 5

Good use of me-time

If this new me-time is to contribute to making you a happier mum,
then what you do with the time is important. Sitting down to watch
TV, for example, can be restful but it won't make you any happier.
In fact, if you are aiming to feel happier, you should cut your
viewing time by at least half. This doesn't mean you *can't* watch
your favourite programmes, but when you find yourself aimlessly
switching channels, switch off instead. Start noticing when you
have the TV on as wallpaper in the background – it's extra noise
and thus extra stress. Switch on to watch something in particular
and then switch off.

Good use of me-time needs to be something that is going to
contribute to your overall well-being and happiness. In general, the
activity you choose should tick one or more of these boxes:

☐	Nurturing	☐	Meditative
☐	Caring	☐	Fun
☐	Calming	☐	Pleasurable
☐	Relaxing	☐	Gladdening
☐	Rewarding	☐	Cheering
☐	Spiritual	☐	Fulfilling

It also needs to be balanced from day to day and week to week. So, you have to balance time for having fun with finding time for being still and calm. Listen to yourself and to what is going on within. Before you became a mum, you probably used to know instinctively what it was you needed for yourself. But now, as your instincts are working at full capacity interpreting your children's needs, you should divert a little energy to thinking about yourself.

Ask yourself:

What is your greatest need today? Do you need to get out there and go dancing and laughing with friends? Or do you need some quiet time to reflect and rebalance?

Ten treats for me-time

And because you've also probably forgotten how to take care of yourself and make good use of me-time, here are ten suggestions for activities and treats:

1. A home pedicure
Ordinarily your feet are probably the last thing you'll find time for and that makes this seem a decadent treat.

First, collect everything you will need:
◆ Some light reading (magazine, paper, cookery book)
◆ Oils (olive and essential)
◆ Soft towel
◆ Pumice stone
◆ Clippers
◆ Tissue (to put nail clippings in)
◆ Nail file

- Moisturiser
- Snuggly socks
- Nail buffer
- Nail polish
- Big glass of red wine or daytime equivalent! Maybe a piece of chocolate?

Run a basin of warm water and add a good squirt of olive oil and a few drops of an essential oil (peppermint or lavender maybe). Soak your feet for ten minutes. Pop the towel on your lap and lift one foot out and pumice it, cut toenails and push back the cuticles with a nail file. Then pop that foot back in the water and do the same with the other foot. After five minutes or so, remove the first foot and lightly dab it dry, then moisturise and put on a sock, then do the same with the other foot (before putting on your sock you could try asking your partner to massage your feet!). Make sure you don't forget to sip your wine/coffee and eat some chocolate while this is taking place.

After twenty minutes or so, take the sock off one foot and buff the nails on that foot. If you don't fancy polish, then that foot is done; put on more moisturiser and put the sock back on. If you want to put polish on, then first put on the basecoat; neaten the other toenails and buff them while this dries, then apply a couple of coats of colour, then more basecoat to hold it in place. Do one foot while the other dries. Doing it this way makes the polish stay as good as new for a couple of weeks. Once the polish is dry, put on more moisturiser and put your socks back on until morning. Obviously, shorten the process as necessary. It's better to do it all in ten minutes than not at all, but please try to find at least ten minutes, interruption free!

2. Phone a friend

Not the friends you see regularly but someone you haven't spoken to for ages perhaps: an old school friend, an old work colleague, an old pre-kids friend? Before you ring, think of four things you'd really like to know about them or from them – jot the questions down. Have you got two interesting things to tell them too? When you ring, check with them whether it's a good time to talk, and if it isn't, book in a time over the next few days.

3. Get some exercise

A key element of making yourself happier is exercise. It's important on so many levels: physical, mental, emotional. Often we are exhausted from getting through the day: cooking, cleaning, washing, ironing, working. Of course, children can be emotionally exhausting with their relentless questions: 'Why, Mum?', 'When, Mum?', 'How, Mum?' It's not surprising that we find it difficult to motivate ourselves to do regular exercise, but the experts have shown that exercise releases all those little happy hormones and endorphins and they firmly suggest that a happiness prescription should include twenty minutes of exercise three times a week. There are some ideas for simple exercise that you can incorporate into your everyday life in Chapter 9, Beating the Blues. Or you can join a class, which is also a way to include some socialising at the same time.

4. Plant something

Gardening helps you feel connected with nature – even briefly. It's about feeling part of something bigger. It means lifting your head out of your own little world. Visit the garden centre and ask what is easy to plant at this time of year. Planting doesn't require lots of equipment or hard work: for example, an impressive selection of lettuces can be grown in a window box. A good idea is to buy a packet of mixed salad seeds that, once grown, can be cut; they grow again, so you get salad all summer from a few plants. Sprinkle thinly and then no thinning will be needed, just harvest as required. Lettuce can also be grown in a grow-bag or can be sown outdoors in winter. As you plant, feel and smell the soil. Look at the little seeds that, with a little care from you, will grow to provide food. Reflect on the miracle of life.

While you're there, can you find an ant and follow it home? Or turn over a big stone to find a family of woodlice? Or, if you can't bear creepy crawlies of any type, put some bread out for the birds and sit quietly. What you need to do is observe and reflect on the busy little lives going on around you: each tiny ant has a place in this world – a job, a life, a daily task.

5. Feel the music

Think of the music you loved as a teenager. Not a sad song that reminds you of your broken heart, but something that you danced to at the school disco. Dig out your old tapes or CDs and find something you haven't listened to for ages . . .

Do you have iTunes or another music download software on your PC? As long as you've got a fairly decent computer, you can download the software free and then download any song for about 70p.

Do you have any of Madonna's stuff, or maybe an eighties' compilation or an Abba album? The choice is yours, but it's got to be something you can dance to. Now, close the curtains and turn up the music as loud as you dare. Dance (as they say) as if no one is watching. You *are* Madonna! Sing at the top of your voice. Keep going for at least four songs. The kids will think you're a bit crazy, but that's OK – it's happy-crazy and they'll love you for it!

Depending on your era, find something from the Bay City Rollers, the Monkees, Abba, Kylie, Bananarama, Duran Duran, Adam and the Ants, or Take That . . .

Here are some of the Netmums' favourite dancing round the sitting room tunes:

- Wham, *Wake Me Up Before You Go Go*
- Duran Duran, *Girls on Film*
- Bon Jovi, *Living on a Prayer*
- Talk Talk, *It's My Life*
- Ultravox, *Vienna*
- Blondie, *Atomic*
- Olivia Newton-John and John Travolta, *Summer Nights*
- Bob Marley, *Three Little Birds*
- Abba, *Waterloo*
- Village People, *YMCA*
- Robbie Williams, *Angels*
- Take That, *Back for Good*
- Queen, *Bohemian Rhapsody*
- The Jacksons, *Can You Feel It?*
- Rose Royce, *Car Wash*
- Bangles, *Manic Monday*
- Dexy's Midnight Runners, *Come On Eileen*
- Queen, *Don't Stop Me Now*
- Katrina and the Waves, *Walking on Sunshine*
- Gloria Gaynor, *I Will Survive*
- Weather Girls, *It's Raining Men*
- Bryan Adams, *Summer of '69*
- The La's, *There She Goes*
- Take That, *Could It Be Magic?*
- ABBA, *SOS*
- B52s, *Love Shack*
- Bananarama, *Venus*
- Boo Radleys, *Wake Up Boo*
- Cyndi Lauper, *Girls Just Wanna Have Fun*
- Joan Jett, *I Love Rock 'n' Roll*

Sing to it, dance to it, walk to it, play it in your car.

6. A relaxing bath

In a straw poll, most mums agreed a real pleasure for a busy mum is a relaxing and peaceful bath followed by clean sheets. Choose your favourite sheets and duvet cover. Maybe spray them with rosewater or a few drops of lavender oil. Run your bath and add your favourite bubble bath or a few drops of lavender oil, and put candles in the bathroom (tea lights work well). Use a hair treatment on your hair (olive oil is wonderful – Joanna Lumley has used it for years, apparently) and maybe a face mask on your face. Maybe bring something to read or some relaxing music into the bathroom, or just close your eyes. Even if the house falls down, don't come out until you have had at least a twenty-minute soak. Rub yourself down with a rough towel and apply heaps of moisturiser or olive or coconut oil.

7. Reflection

Can you find your way to a church, chapel, synagogue or other holy place or building? There is an atmosphere in a holy place that, even if you are not religious, seems to penetrate right through the walls. Spend ten minutes reflecting on the quietness, calmness and peace. Try to empty your mind of daily chatter and noise and busy thoughts. Imagine the peace seeping into and through you. If there are candles, light one, leaving a little light shining behind you and take the peace with you. With every breath, breathe in the peace and breathe out the tension.

8. A new magazine

A new magazine is such a small but significant pleasure. Find half an hour today to sit with a magazine (a trashy gossip mag is great escapism, but if that's not your thing maybe one on fashion or interiors or food). You need peace and quiet – and if you can have peace and quiet on a fine day in the garden that's even better. If you can't afford a new magazine, the charity shops usually have a decent selection, but with many magazines on sale for £1 do try to pick one up.

With your magazine, you need a really good coffee or favourite drink. Brew fresh coffee just for you. Use your posh china – a proper cup and saucer. Have a biscuit or two or slice of cake with NO guilt! Or try this superb iced coffee treat:

- Take a heaped teaspoon of instant coffee.
- Add enough hot water to cover.
- Stir until dissolved.
- Add a good-sized scoop of vanilla ice cream and a mug of ice cold milk.
- Use a blender, mixer or whisk to whizz it round until the ice cream has melted and it's all frothy.
- Pour it into a long glass and sweeten to taste.
- The grown-up equivalent of a milkshake, it's delicious.

9. Personal grooming

Someone recently described happiness as the forty-eight hours after waxing! Whatever your take on hair removal, it always feels good afterwards, so plan a time for it. Book a wax, or get a new razor blade, or a tube of hair remover and get to it: legs, underarms, bikini line. Now sort out your eyebrows: get them plucked, or threaded, or ask a friend or do it yourself. A good tip is to line a pencil in a straight line up the side of your nose: where it reaches your eyebrows is where they should start. Now move the pencil to a diagonal line from the bottom of your nose to the outer corner of your eye socket and that's where it should finish.

10. Go out for coffee . . .

. . . without any children. If you like, take a newspaper, magazine, crossword or Sudoku puzzle. Order whatever you fancy – a cappuccino, or latte and maybe a muffin. Find a nice comfy chair and sink into it; stretch out your legs. Take a deep breath in and out and release all your tension. Spend a little time enjoying the moment being an adult in the adult world. People-watch for a bit. Stay there for at least twenty minutes. Thank the waiter or waitress with a smile and put something in the tips jar. Then go back to reality.

And finally . . . keeping up appearances

You don't need to buy into the myth that mums should look glamorous and fabulous. Nor should you put on a mask and pretend you feel great when you don't. Keeping up appearances is about keeping up your self-esteem and believing you are worth it. You are a woman as well as a mum and you can still feel beautiful if and when you need to. It's about feeling OK about yourself and giving yourself a little confidence boost.

Here are a few tips that won't change your life but might lift your mood a little:

♦ Keep a bottle of fake tan to hand and apply a little at night to your face and neck every couple of days before you do your teeth at night. It takes away that first depressing look at a tired face in the bathroom mirror in the morning. Just a quick application at night and you'll find yourself looking in the mirror thinking, 'Actually, I don't look too bad!'

♦ Invest in a pair of eyelash curlers – you can pick them up in the chemist's for under a fiver. Thirty seconds on each set of lashes can make your eyes look wider and brighter.

♦ A good-hair day can make all the difference between holding your head high and flicking your hair back with confidence or sticking it up in a scrunchy and keeping your head down. A good haircut can really help, as can taking Omega-3 fish oils, which are great for the hair and skin as well as for your brain. For emergencies (of the 'Hi, I'm just round the corner, shall I pop round for a coffee?' kind or the 'I'm late for work' kind) keep a bottle of dry shampoo handy (you just squirt it on and brush it out), then tie all your hair back except the fringe or front section, and wash that bit and blow-dry it. You'll have that just-stepped-out-of-the-salon look in five minutes flat!

♦ Update your make-up bag: there are lots of very cheap cosmetics that mimic the designer brands brilliantly. An inexpensive new lip gloss, or eyeliner in a different colour, or nail varnish can give you a real lift: you get that buzz from getting something new for you, and it costs only a couple of pounds.

♦ Lots of mums tell us that they don't buy any new clothes, as they'd rather spend their money on their children. Well, no one *needs* fancy clothing, but little children need it even less. If you've stopped buying new clothes for yourself, do ask yourself why.

Ask yourself:

Why don't you care about the way you look?

If you are thinking right now that you really don't care about how you look, your children are more important and that side of your life had changed for ever, then it might be worth asking yourself why you feel that way.

♦ Have you lost so much self-esteem that you feel a little effort won't do any good and that you'd need full-scale cosmetic surgery to make any real difference at this stage?

♦ Could it be that you don't feel you are worth it?

♦ Or do you feel that if you don't make any effort you'll be somehow more invisible?

Ask the Netmums:

Is looking good important to you?

Looking good is very important to me – it helps me to feel like Lindsay and not just Jasmyn's mummy. It's about who I am and is part of me. I've recently slimmed down to a size 10 – after the little one's birth I was up to an 18 . . . so now I can wear the trendy clothes I've wanted to for ages. Although I've always spent a lot on make-up (Dior or Mac), it makes me feel that little bit special having it . . . Walking out the door looking great and feeling healthy pushing my gorgeous little girl is a fab feeling and has helped to keep away the blues.

Lindsay, Ellesmere Port, mum to Jasmyn, 15 months

I've just stopped bothering (nearly) completely. I used to wear make-up every time I left the house, and generally tried to look nice. Now I would bother only if I was going out-out (you know, after kiddies' bedtime, with other grown-ups), but because this doesn't actually happen, I haven't worn make-up in over three months. I was never fussy about my hair, it's too straight to do anything, but I stopped dyeing it when I got pregnant and haven't dyed it since.

I haven't minded being a slob, because most days the only people to see me are my son and his father, but now that I'm starting university I have begun to worry about my appearance more. I have been thinking of dyeing my hair again, and wondering whether I should wear make-up or not. I know these are quite silly worries, but I haven't had to make an impression on others in years and I do worry about not fitting in.

Clothes shopping is quite a strange and rare experience now. Instead of buying something for myself, I end up blowing my budget on my little one. I just don't know how to shop for myself any more; I'm not even sure what kind of clothes I like or don't like these days. I'm so out of fashion. . .
Jutta, North London, mum to Aki, 18 months

I don't bother at all any more – my son is much more important. Any spare money gets spent on him rather than buying clothes and make-up for me. When I absolutely have to buy clothes with no way of getting around it, I get the cheapest things possible – it's just not important to me any more.
Fran, Southeast London, mum to Benjamin, 14 months

I have never really been into expensive make-up or designer clothes; my make-up bag mainly consists of Rimmel or Maybelline, and before children I always used to live in jeans and shop on the high street, so that is still the same really. However, I do like to look the best that I can and it makes me feel good about myself. I do like to buy new clothes; sadly, that is not always possible, as the kids always need something. I never leave the house without straightening my hair and without my make-up on.
Sam, Wolverhampton, mum to Alex, 9, Hollie, 7 and Lewis, 4

I do bother with myself and don't usually slob about in trackies and T-shirts, as I want to look nice and feel good. I'm not a follower of fashion, as I am on the large side, but I do my hair and wear perfume and a trace of make-up each day, and although I don't wear heels I do try to wear smart and trendy clothes for my size. My husband says I

always look nice and I think it is important that you don't give up your identity, as you can still be you, as well as your little treasures' mummy.
Wendy, Harrow, mum to Glen, 6 and Greg, 5

I was wondering the other day if I had finally let myself go . . . too far . . . when I saw a very yummy mummy at baby gym looking at my unshaved legs with a look of barely concealed horror. I figured that it's approaching autumn, so I'll be back in tights soon anyway!

I have to be reasonably smart on the three days I work, but on the other days I tend to slob in my oldest scruffy clothes. I rarely go to the hairdresser – I just snip at my fringe when it gets in my eyes! To be honest, though, I've never been into fashion and make-up anyway – I think I'm glammed up if I put a bit of powder and foundation on.
Sue, Leeds, mum of three boys and a girl, 13, 11, 7, and 20 months

It's really important to me to look good. I love clothes and enjoy shopping for them. I wouldn't dream of going out of the house without my make-up on (I would scare everyone). I like my hair to be nice too. I've always been like that, though. I need to make the best of what I've got, which isn't much.
Sara, Dunfermline, mum to Rachel, 6 and Lara, 4

I am a thirty-three-year-old mum to two children. I always try to make an effort, and I am very good at shopping for bargains. I enjoy having new clothes each season but like lots for my money, so I don't mind if they are from Matalan or Asda. Every day I like to have clean hair and always wear

make-up and perfume. I am not a naturally confident and assertive person, so this helps to make me feel better. I am not vain at all and don't like my body much, but I do try to make the most of myself to feel good and happy without spending too much. My children's clothes often cost more than mine, especially shoes! I dress just as I did before I became a mummy and don't think that should change. We are all different – you should just wear what you are happy in!
Gina, Lancashire, mum to Amelia, 6 and William, 3

Most of my money goes on my kids these days. As long as my clothes are clean, and I have brushed hair when leaving the house, I am happy. But, yes, sometimes buying something new makes me feel good; for example, I went to a Christening last weekend and bought a new top that gave me slightly more confidence.
Jacqui, Peterborough, mum to Liam, 7, Zack, 5 and Ellis, 10 months

I think it's important to look nice, as when you feel you look nice it can give you an improved self-confidence and this will be reflected when your kids look at you. I don't think my clothes have changed – if anything, they've improved, as I want my daughter to grow up being proud to have a mum like me. The only thing I do wear a lot is trainers or flat shoes as they're more practical running around after a child. I think too many people have kids and lose themselves, which can lead to them being depressed. Don't forget who you are: you're not just a mum, you're a person. Have respect for yourself. You feeling good about yourself will help others around you feel that way too.
Wendy, Northampton, mum to Caitlin, 3

I love getting dressed up, but I also think getting obsessed with it is a bit superficial. I will always put the little one's important needs before mine, which means if push comes to shove I'll go out looking very slummy mummy. Whenever possible (and certainly for work) I will do the necessary, but I'd like her to grow up realising that women have things between their ears that matter more than designer jeans and eyeliner.

Clare, Sheffield, mum to Olivia, 14 months

Don't worry about fashion . . . just be clean! Sounds easy, but with toddlers around your ankles all day it's very easy to go out with greasy hair 'just this once', but it's a slippery slope. You always feel better when you've had a shower too!

Bethan, Swansea, mum to Abigail, 2 and Oliver, 1

9 Beating the Blues

Your children are healthy and happy, your husband is kind and (mostly) helpful, you've got a roof over your head and food in the fridge, and all is well with your world. And yet . . . you feel a bit on edge. For no apparent reason, you feel anxious and agitated and you can't seem to get anything finished. You feel permanently tired and headachy. You're beginning to wonder if there is something wrong with your health. You're snappy and grumpy at home and don't feel much like seeing your friends or socialising. You overreact to the smallest thing your child does and then feel awful guilt for shouting.

If this sounds like you, you could well be suffering from excess stress or depression, and you certainly aren't the only one. In our increasingly fast world, many of us are having trouble keeping up.

Netmums did some research in 2005 and found that we are three times more likely to have post-natal depression than our mums. So, despite all our mod cons and more choice, we are unhappier and more stressed than our parents' generation.

Suggestions for why this is include:
– Our generation is less likely than ever before to live near our parents and extended family. We are lonelier and more isolated than our parents were.
– We wanted the freedom to choose to work, but ironically, having achieved that, many of us now don't have a choice – we have to work to pay the bills. So more of us than ever are living the stressful life of a working mum.
– We are bombarded with media images of beautiful, thin, fashionable have-it-all mothers and perfect, expensively dressed children living in beautifully coordinated homes. The reality is sure to be a let-down!
– We have learned to believe that *stuff* makes us happy – the more we get, the more we buy, the better and happier our lives will be. Only it doesn't work . . .

Does any of this apply to you? If we are honest, we have probably all tried at some point to be A Perfect Mum to show our family, friends and the world in general that we have got a handle on this whole motherhood thing. We can keep a tidy home, look nice, have great kids, great marriages, and a career – nope, no problems here! Many mums quickly realise that they've bought into a lie and get back to reality fast, but others keep going, keep trying to achieve this impossible goal. They retain the belief that to let go of any of it, to admit to not being perfect, would be to fail as a mother – and to fail as a mother is surely the ultimate failure. So they push themselves ever harder. They keep their foot flat on the accelerator long after they've got stuck in the mud, wheels spinning; rather than moving on, they get more and more stuck.

Symptoms of stress or depression

Here is a list of symptoms that can apply to stress or depression. See if any of them apply to you:

+ Feeling overwhelmed and unable to cope
+ Feeling a constant underlying sense of anxiety, maybe escalating into panic attacks
+ Being easily 'set off' and difficult to calm down
+ Feeling guilty about everything, especially about being such a bad mother
+ Constantly feeling tired, with no energy
+ Having problems sleeping –– not being able to get to sleep or waking in the early hours and not being able to get back to sleep
+ Crying a lot, often over the smallest things or for no reason at all
+ Not being able to eat or over-eating
+ Feeling you are wearing a mask: always putting on a cheerful front when in reality you feel anything but
+ Feeling emotionally disconnected from life, as though you are playing out a role rather than living in the moment
+ Being overly anxious and over-protective of your children, maybe experiencing strange, frightening thoughts or visions popping into your head about awful things happening
+ Having a lack of motivation to get up and do anything or a fanatical need to get everything done and get on top of everything, e.g. frantically making lists, or even a combination

of the two: making the lists but feeling incapable of doing anything about them, thus leading to further anxiety

♦ Having to have things done in a certain way and not being able to let it go, even occasionally (for example, 'The kitchen floor must be washed every day with antibacterial cleaner and the sofa cushions and curtains must be straight the way I like them')

♦ Having difficulty concentrating, say on a book or film or even on a conversation

♦ Feeling lonely and isolated; perhaps feeling rejected by friends, family, even your partner and your baby or children

♦ Experiencing physical aches and pains, such as headaches, stomach pains or blurred vision, and worrying that it is something serious or terminal

Physical symptoms may include:
♦ A dry throat and constant thirst
♦ An upset tummy with a regular touch of diarrhoea
♦ Urinating more than usual
♦ No interest in sex
♦ Times when your heart seems to pound in your chest
♦ Muscle aches and pains
♦ Dizzy spells
♦ Shakes or tremors
♦ Feeling hot or cold
♦ Sweating
♦ Frequent cold sores or mouth ulcers
♦ A constant anxious knot just below your ribcage

If you recognise yourself in two or three of these emotional symptoms and are experiencing any of the physical symptoms, it would seem likely that you are suffering from the symptoms of bad stress or possibly even depression.

Stress or depression?

Of course, feeling temporarily stressed because you are moving house or have a deadline coming up doesn't mean you have depression. Stress, in itself, isn't always a bad thing; it's a normal physical reaction designed to stimulate our 'fight or flight' response. Our ancestors needed to be watchful for signs of a predator who fancied them for dinner or be on the outlook for a rival tribe on the attack. At the first sign of danger, the body produces a burst of hormones that makes your breathing get faster, your heart speed up and your muscles tense: your body is ready to fight the attacker or run as fast as possible from the predator, hence the term 'fight or flight'.

We can make positive use of this stress reaction: a bit of adrenaline can help us to think clearly and more quickly before an exam or job interview. It can help you as a mum to react quickly if you see your three year old halfway up a ladder or on the edge of a pond. But when we are producing a heavy duty stress response to a spilt milk bottle or an overturned plate of spaghetti; or when our 'fight' mechanism springs into action at a tantruming toddler or a husband reading the paper instead of washing up; or when we want to run out the door, get in the car and drive away from unmade beds and breakfast chaos . . . this is perhaps when we need to look at our stress levels and decide whether we are suffering from bad stress or a bit of depression.

For mums, it can often be quite tricky to sort out what is causing the psychological muddle we find ourselves in. Are you stressed by the constant demands of babies and young children? Is your stress caused by exhaustion? Are you depressed because you can't keep on top of everything, or can you not keep on top of everything because you are depressed? Do stress and exhaustion lead to depression? Is it all caused by the huge hormonal upheaval of pregnancy and childbirth? Or is it something to do with those issues from your childhood? Or is it because you've got so little help and support? Maybe it's just the overwhelming life-changing event of becoming a mother.

The truth is: it is probably a bit of all of these. But the interesting thing for us is that the things we can do to help ourselves feel better are the same regardless of the cause.

Bad stress

For many mums who are suffering from stress, it is not simply enough to look at one specific issue. If you have been neglecting yourself for quite some time, it may be that you are suffering from overstress. Basically, this means that you are always on alert. Your body has forgotten how to switch off the panic button. Pretty much anything and everything that doesn't go entirely according to plan causes you to feel stressed. By now, you are, in fact, *overreacting* to much of what happens.

This is an impossible situation for a mum with young children, because, as we all know, nothing ever goes according to plan. It is only by learning the art of going with the flow of life with young children that we can hope to be happy mums. If you are overstressed, it means that your body isn't able to regulate itself. It gets so used to being on permanent alert that it never gets the signal that it is OK to relax, that it's OK to pull back those fighting hormones and let the relaxing, calming hormones in to do their job.

There are techniques to deal with stress and they do work. We need to send our mind and body some very strong messages. But to do this, it does mean making it a priority in your life to lower your stress levels. It is crucial that you find time in your life for this.

Too much stress puts a strain on your heart and can lead to heart disease and high blood pressure. It can lead to an unhappy home for you, your partner and your children.

Children are very sensitive to atmosphere and moods. They use you as a mirror and they will mimic your stress levels, which in turn will lead them to feel on edge and irritable and, in time, this could affect their mental and physical well-being. If you don't have the motivation to do it for yourself (it's very hard to find the extra energy when you are already exhausted), do it for *them*.

Ask yourself:

What are your flashpoints?

Keep a stress diary for a few days – a week if you can. Keep it with you and try to write a line or so every hour or two. Note the day and the time. Include your physical world (where you are, who you're with, what's going on) and your internal world (is something or someone on your mind? are you tired?). Mark your stress level out of 10. Give yourself a 2 or 3 out of 10 for when you are relaxed and maybe gently pottering, a 6 or 7 when you feel a little uneasy, and a 9 or 10 when you feel like screaming or crying!

After a week, can you look back and see what has been going on? What are your triggers or flashpoints? It could be something obviously big in your life, such as a bereavement or something that happened in your childhood, or it can be something seemingly trivial, such as a broken washing machine or uneaten food, or thinking about a certain person or event. The point is: if it is causing you to feel stressed, anxious or depressed, then it isn't trivial. You need to recognise it as a 'stressor' and look at what is going on around it. Is it a particular time of day? Are you usually more stressed in the evenings when you are tired, for example? Or is it a particular situation or a certain person or event?

A note about quick fixes

It's very tempting to look for the quick fix. Cigarettes, alcohol, packets of chocolate biscuits, lots of coffee or caffeine drinks all offer a quick fix. For a moment, or maybe a bit longer, we feel better. We feel comforted, relaxed or in control. Isn't that massively tempting, especially when we haven't got the time or money to book into The Priory? It's no wonder huge numbers of people are self-medicating with quick fixes. But deep down we know it doesn't really work. Of course, there is nothing wrong with a couple of glasses of wine or a biscuit with your coffee, but it's when you *need* it that you should look at what you are using it for.

Ask yourself:

Do you feel satisfied in yourself about the way you use alcohol or food or cigarettes? Or do you sometimes feel ashamed, guilty or concerned? If so, can you commit to using some other techniques for stress management such as the ones outlined in this chapter?

Sadly, as with all things in life, there are no quick fixes. Having said that, the good techniques for stress relief are enjoyable in themselves: not only do they reduce stress but they will make you feel more positive, optimistic, energetic and fundamentally happier.

Ask the Netmums:

How do you cope with stress?

My other half will take over, while I go and have a few minutes to myself to de-stress. I do the same for him if he's got them and is getting stressed. It seems easier to deal with when you can walk away and know the little ones are safe. My favourite way to de-stress is to cook. My other half can tell if I had a bad day, because he gets a lovely home-cooked meal or fancy cake I've made. An ideal way for me to relax is to spend the day cooking for a dinner party or making/preparing food for parties!

Jenny, Canterbury, mum to Benjamin, 3 and James, 18 months

When I get stressed, I shout at the boys and then cry because I feel awful for shouting at them for doing what kids do. I then go for a bath and take a book or magazine with me for half an hour's peace (either while hubby looks after them or they are in bed). If it's too early for a bath and bed and hubby is around, I tend to leave the boys with him and pop to my mum's for half an hour to get my act together. She doesn't really understand about post-natal depression and tells me I should control myself and not shout or get stressed (she means it in a nice way though).

Michelle, Rochester, mum to Harry, 3 and Charlie, 16 months

When I'm stressed I:
– Scream into a pillow.
– Go for a walk.
– Phone my friends for a chat.
– Take it out on my other half!
– Have a nice, long, hot bubble bath and read.
– Put my music on full blast (so I can't hear the kids, as it's
   usually their fault!)
Leigh, Manchester, mum to Tom, 12 and Jack, 4

I get out of the house with the pushchair (generally
guaranteed to keep the boys quiet; well, Samuel anyway).
Alternatively, I eat chocolate, but shouting, crying and
swearing inside my head all work well too!
*Helen, East Dorset, mum to Thomas, 2 and Samuel, 10
months*

I use self-hypnosis tapes by Paul McKenna. They are quite
fantastic and work a treat (apart from the one that claims
to make me thin – that still hasn't worked!)
Claudia, Bedford, mum to Sophia, 5 and Mia, 3

If I'm stressed, I can't work so I stop everything and run a hot
bubble bath and spend up to four hours in the bath,
topping up lots while I read a full book. Sex is good too –
totally works out all the mental kinks!
Donna, Rotherham, mum to Samuel, 5 and Emma, 3

I scoop everyone up and head for the great outdoors –
even if it is raining, we get on wellies and macs and twirl our
umbrellas. Even if everyone is still crying or whinging, it
always sounds less piercing in the fresh air! My lifeline when

I was a new mum with a colicky baby was to make a beeline for places with very few people around and stomp with a buggy, and more often than not we would arrive home less wound up than when we left. If it was a magic day, Hannah would even be asleep, so I could follow it up with a cup of tea and a flop, ready for the next bit!

If it is the wrong time of year and too cold or wet, I switch the mood by playing loud music (Scissor Sisters seem to work or Robbie!) and dance around the living room – anyone cross usually forgets why and we jig to the music and cheer up. We bounce wildly and forget our woes. I may not be able to get away with this one for too much longer, as I seem to have developed a mum-dance despite being a groovy chick in my pre-mummy days!

If I am stressed for reasons other than the kids, then I talk, talk, talk. I pick up the phone or grab a friend/hubby/kind-looking old lady at the bus stop and talk it out. I always feel better afterwards, even if we haven't found the answer. If it is too late to chat, I email or write it down; often I don't send my maudlin messages, but I feel like I have got it all off my chest anyway and it does feel better.

Sometimes at 'flashpoints' (i.e. those short stressy times when you are trying to get out of the house and someone has kicked someone else, someone has pooed on the carpet and there is only one shoe), I stop what I am doing, abandon everyone (safely) and go into a room and take a wee moment to calm myself before I blow. I breathe deeply and shake myself out and re-compose. Once I even strapped everyone in the car and went back inside to chill for a minute and returned as a sane mummy again!

Nicola, Edinburgh, mum to Hannah, 5 and Feena, 3

In no particular order, as it depends on location, circum-stances and time of day . . .

1. Loud music always helps – something I can sing along to and dance like a fool. The kids join in, which lifts their spirits and stops them bickering too. The Jam is our current favourite. Or something uplifting and 'nice', such as Jack Johnson or Corinne Bailey Rae.
2. Play the piano . . . loudly!
3. Sit on the kitchen floor and shout, 'I need a cuddle!' They all come running and we end up in a heap, laughing and kissing.
4. Phone my best friend and have a good mutual rant!
5. Go for a fast walk by the river.
6. Rescue Remedy and a cuppa.
7. Salutation to the Sun or any inverted yoga pose.
8. Force my shoulders down and back, straighten my back, swing my arms around a few times and deep breathe through the nose (Pranayama).
9. Throw my toys out of the pram!

Christine, Kingston, mum to Isabelle, 8, Aimee, 6 and Ethan, 3

I have a cry in the bathroom – the only place I can go without being interrupted! But I have been known to have a good sob without a care for whoever is around when I'm really stressed. Once, when I was expecting Maisy and trying to organise our house move from London to Warwick, I burst into tears at work when someone asked how it was all going! I do tend to recognise how stressed I am only when the tears start flowing. Having a bath in complete peace with some nice scented candles and classical music is my other nicer stress buster, although quite often I might have a little sob in there too! Think I might be off to do that one this evening – today has been a bit of a stressful one!

Caroline, Warwickshire, mum to Abigail, 5 and Maisy, 3

A stress-busting toolbox

This tool box contains a selection of techniques or tools you can use to help yourself feel better. It might be that you need a certain tool to help you fix a specific problem. Or it might be that you need to use a combination of tools over a long period . . . It depends on you and also on how long you have been neglecting your emotional well-being.

The tools that can help you deal with stress and depression are:

1. Talking
2. Relaxing
3. Exercising
4. Eating well

1. Talking

Have you ever noticed how the old-fashioned sayings, expressions and beliefs have a way of resurfacing? Mums were giving their children cod liver oil long before we had heard of Omega-3 fish oils! Well, here's another one: 'A problem shared is a problem halved' or another: 'No man [Mum!] is an island.' We need other people. However tough we think we are, we do need to open up and tell other people about how we are feeling. The problem is that one of the symptoms of stress or depression is to put up barriers and close ourselves off from our emotions and other people. We put up these barriers in the hope of protecting ourselves or to avoid burdening others, but they end up keeping the problem locked up inside. It can be scary letting our deep-seated thoughts, worries and anxieties out of their box but ultimately, however well hidden they are, they will stay there inside us. We need to look at whether we can get those worries out in the open, have a really good look at them, examine them from all angles, talk them over with someone else and use their sense of perspective when ours is out of proportion. Studies have found that talking to people about the things that concern you actually changes the way the brain works and combats depression and anxiety. But who can you talk to?

Friends and family

Most of us aren't lucky enough to have a close-knit group of friends living locally whom we can share all our worries with, but most of us do have someone we can talk to. It's often that we don't feel able or willing to open up, as that makes us vulnerable. It also means admitting we aren't perfect and our lives aren't perfect. We worry that if we show ourselves as we really are, we will be less lovable. The truth is that no one has a perfect life and by admitting that and being open about your worries, you will appear more human, more real and approachable and thus more, rather than less, lovable.

Choose someone you feel you can talk to – ideally choose two people so that you can spread the load a little. The obvious choices are your mum and your partner, but if your mum isn't around and your partner isn't great at emotional stuff, look a bit further afield: a friend's mum perhaps, a neighbour, even? Older people, especially older mums, have usually been through a lot and are often full of wisdom and good advice. And they may have the time to spend with you. Generally, people are pleased to be asked for help. If someone approached you and said they were having a hard time and needed a sounding board and asked if you could spare half an hour, would you be happy to help? Of course! If it makes you more comfortable, ask them if you can speak to them in confidence and if they will guarantee you that confidentiality. Give others the opportunity to help you.

A professional

There are many advantages in talking to a professional. Professionals are trained to guide you and advise you and, of course, there is a wonderful freedom in having up to a full hour to talk about yourself without having to worry about whether you are boring the other person.

In a very simplistic way there are two approaches to counselling, although the best counsellors probably use a combination of both.

Psychotherapy

Psychotherapy is about understanding what makes you tick: what experiences in your life led you to this place and how you really feel about things. This is useful if you have had a traumatic experience in childhood or later life, such as an abusive or alcoholic partner or parent, a parent absent from your life either physically or emotionally, or being badly bullied at school. Or you might want to explore much more recent events, such as a traumatic childbirth, coming to terms with a special needs child, the recent death of a parent or friend, or a relationship breakdown.

Many mums agree that when we become mothers, especially for the first time, the impact of having this helpless, defenceless child dependent on us can cause a huge emotional surge that can bring to the surface many deeply buried emotions and experiences. It could be that something you thought you had suppressed within yourself long ago has resurfaced and needs to be dealt with. A counsellor will help you look at these things and find a way to make them feel safe.

Cognitive Behaviour Therapy (CBT)

If there isn't a 'big issue' that is causing your stress or depression, a course in CBT can be hugely effective. CBT helps you to challenge your thoughts and retrain your brain patterns to think in different, more positive ways.

And a recent study found that in women with post-natal depression a course of cognitive-behavioural counselling is as effective as an antidepressant drug.[1]

Ask yourself:

The next time you feel upset, stressed or worried about something, can you stop and note down what your thoughts are? Can you challenge what you were thinking and find a different way of thinking about what's happening? Here is a simple CBT exercise you can try to give you an idea of how it works.

Are you thinking something critical about yourself?
Are you thinking, 'I'm a terrible mother and a total failure'? Ask yourself how someone else might view the situation. Would they see a failure, or a mum with a nice house, a lovely, clean, happy baby and a good relationship?

Are you predicting the future instead of facing it when it happens?
'My child won't eat, therefore he won't grow properly.' Ask yourself, 'What is the evidence for that?' Is your baby gaining weight? What does his growth chart say?

Are you telling yourself how you ought to behave?
Do you use the words 'should', 'ought' and 'must' a lot? For example: 'I must clean the house.' Ask yourself, 'Why should

(1) Appleby, L., Warner, R., Whitton, A. and Faragher, B., *A controlled study of fluoxetine and cognitive-behavioural counselling in the treatment of post-natal depression*, 1997 (BMJ 314: 932-6)

I? What will happen if I don't?' Perhaps it's time to change your expectations.

Are you considering the worst-case scenario?
'If I go out, the baby will probably scream, I'll have a panic attack and make a total fool of myself and won't be able to cope.' What is the evidence to support the thought? Did you make a total fool of yourself last time . . . and, if so, in whose eyes? Did anyone notice? Does it really matter?

Try to step outside and look in on the situation.
What would someone who cares about you say to you? What advice would you give to someone else in this situation?

How to find a counsellor

Your doctor can refer you to a counsellor and you can have some talking therapy on the NHS. Sadly, in many areas, waiting lists are long. You could also go privately, and again your doctor may be able to refer you to someone he knows and trusts locally. For a psychotherapist or clinical psychologist, you can expect to pay anywhere between £50–£80 an hour. Yes, it's a lot, but if it's your health and happiness and that of your family at stake, can you find the money? If it was a physical illness that could be cured with £1,000, could you find the money? Just because it is a mental health issue doesn't make it less important. If the waiting list for the NHS is very long in your area and you can't afford to go private, your health visitor is a good alternative. Phone or call in to book an appointment. Many health visitors are trained in counselling skills, and all health visitors are trained to listen.

There are many very well-meaning counsellors out there. But do remember that a counsellor can be so called after completing a one-year correspondence course, whereas a clinical psychologist has been through a rigorous training programme: a four-year degree in psychology followed by a further three years studying clinical psychology. So check the counsellor's background and qualifications: a poor counsellor stirring up deep-rooted feelings and emotions and not knowing what to do with them can cause more harm than good.

Not only do you need a well-qualified and experienced professional, but you also need someone you can work well with. That is impossible to define, but it is similar to the relationship with your doctor, perhaps. Any doctor can write you a prescription, but with some doctors you feel you can tell them anything and just visiting them makes you feel better. In this case, they are much more likely to write you the right prescription. So it is with counsellors. There are lots of mums who have sought help from a counsellor, not got on with them and decided counselling in general isn't for them. So if you fall at the first hurdle, be prepared to try again with a different counsellor.

Here are some points you might also like to consider and investigate before starting to work with a counsellor:
- Is the counsellor qualified (i.e. have they reached diploma or degree level)?
- Is the counsellor insured to work with clients?
- You could ask to see his or her certification and up-to-date insurance documents.
- Does the counsellor have regular supervision from a qualified

supervisor (approximately one to two hours per month)?
- Does the counsellor belong to a recognised organisation, such as the British Association for Counselling and Psychotherapy (BACP), UK Register of Counsellors (UKRC), UK Council for Psychotherapy (UKCP), or another similar body?
- When and where does he or she see clients?
- How much does he or she charge, how do you pay, and is there a reduction for those on low wages?
- Does he or she offer a free, or reduced, introductory session?
- What are the arrangements for holidays and cancelled or missed appointments?

On meeting the counsellor, ask yourself if you like him or her. Do you feel comfortable in his or her presence and do you think that he or she is able to meet your needs? You do not have to make up your mind on the spot; ask for time to think about continuing. Let the counsellor know if it is possible to contact you, and how you would like to be contacted (e.g. telephone, mobile or letter), and if messages can be left for you anywhere in case of late cancellations, etc. Finally, remember that if you are not happy or you are unsure about the way a counsellor is working with you, tell him or her. However, if you are happy with the way you've worked together, then pass your recommendation on to any friend in need.

Home-Start
Home-Start is a national charity with local branches all over the country. It offers a befriending scheme for mums (or dads) with children under five who are struggling with life, for whatever reason, and need a supportive and non-judgemental friend. Basically, they are friends in need. They'll match you up with a volunteer. This will usually be an older or more experienced mum who has been through the tough years of having young children

and wants to help. She'll come to see you probably once a week and talk, play with the children and generally be a friend for as long as you need her. While Home-Start does not have a magic formula to take all the problems away, parents say that having a friend to confide in, to cry with, to laugh with and to talk to can make all the difference.

> **Phone the national Home-Start line on 0800 068 63 68 to find details of your local Home-Start branch (there are 337 throughout the country). They'll have a chat with you and try to match you with someone suitable, someone they think you'll get on with.**

Ask the Netmums:
Did you find Home-Start helpful?

I had no problems after the birth of my son James, but six weeks after my daughter Charlotte was born, I was already starting to suffer from depression. I just didn't seem to have the energy to do anything, and would sit around the house feeling guilty for not keeping on top of things. After my maternity leave finished, I returned to work, but was eventually signed off sick. The doctor was sympathetic, but I was put on a long waiting list for counselling and given anti-depressants.

Learning to look after two small children seemed like the most difficult thing in the world and, as we'd recently moved house, I didn't have many friends locally. I asked my health visitor for ideas and she suggested Home-Start. I wasn't really interested in 'therapy' and couldn't afford to pay for counselling anyway, but I thought that having someone to talk to once a week would be nice . . .

I can't tell you what a difference it made. Wendy came round each week and we played with the children. Occasionally she'd ask how I was feeling, but really she was just someone to share the children with, and to chat to. I would always look forward to Thursday mornings. Over time, I found I gained confidence, and started to make new friends and gradually recovered from the depression. When I was happy to go it alone, Wendy stopped visiting and is now helping other families – I owe her so much. Home-Start really is about being a friend to you. It's for 'normal' people who need some extra support . . . after all, for many people, bringing up young children can be the most difficult time in our lives.

Sally, Watford, mum to James, 10 and Charlotte, 7

I have two sons and Home-Start was initially suggested by my health visitor following the birth of my second son, when I experienced severe post-natal illness. I was very nervous when Jackie first came, but we hit it off very quickly. The first eight months following Luke's birth were really, really hard, but Jackie was always there. I suffered from hallucinations and Jackie was often with me when this happened. I'd feel too guilty to tell my family and believed I was going mad, but Jackie would comfort me and reassure me that things were OK and it would pass. I was suicidal at times and I'm sure she saved my life on a number of occasions just by being there.

The children know and love her and now see her as part of our family. She was also wonderful with my husband and was really the only person to ask how *he* was through all of this. There are not many people you can bare your soul to and really trust that they won't let you down. Jackie was always honest with me and provided me with lots of reassurance.

I'm so much better now. I am off anti-depressants and Jackie no longer visits, but we do keep in touch. I am now a member of Home-Start's management committee and try to help in any way I can, because of what they've done for me.

Tania

2. Relaxing

Our body and minds are so closely interlinked that it is very hard to have a stressed-out mind inside a completely relaxed body. Relaxation exercises imprint a feeling of relaxation on your body and mind. Basically, you're learning a new habit. Remember that they are called relaxation *exercises* and an exercise means something that has to be worked at. So you must work at relaxing – not just sit in front of the telly – but it can be the most pleasurable 'work' you've ever done.

Guided relaxation

Guided relaxation means having someone you can listen to who guides you through the relaxation process. Generally speaking, this is more effective than doing it yourself, because you can rely on the other voice and completely free up your mind to concentrate on the business at hand.

There is a lovely series from Dr Jack Gibson, a pioneer of deep relaxation and hypnosis. Dr Gibson worked as a surgeon during the First World War in the hospitals of the Emergency Medical Service. He learned to use deep relaxation on soldiers needing operations whose bodies were too deeply shocked to take the strong general anaesthetic of those days. He developed and perfected his skills and continued to work with patients with stress, depression or addictions long after he retired from being a surgeon. In 1969, he launched a record, 'How to Stop Smoking', which went straight to number one for six weeks, depriving The Beatles of the top spot! He continued to work with patients until his recent death in Dublin at the age of 94. He has left behind a series of excellent tapes and CDs, which can be bought online at www.drjackgibson.com.

Paul McKenna is a more modern-day practitioner with global success, and has produced tapes and CDs on relaxation and stress control as well as weight loss and stopping smoking.

There are many other good relaxation tapes and CDs, and it's a question of finding one that suits you, with a voice and an accent you like. Many libraries carry tapes or might be willing to order one for you, or try local bookstores and online.

A simple relaxation exercise

Find a comfortable place, ideally sitting up in a good armchair. Don't cross your legs, and have your feet flat on the floor, without shoes.

Breathe deeply in and out a few times. Say to yourself on the in-breath, 'I need to relax', and on the out-breath, 'I will relax'. Clear your head. Push aside any thoughts that enter your head the way a car window wiper pushes the rain aside.

Start at your little toe on your right foot and relax it, then the next toe and the next, until your five toes are relaxed. Move slowly up the bones in your foot, feeling each one relax, deeply relax and sink into the floor.

It can be helpful to imagine a white line starting in your toes and slowly, slowly moving through the inside of your feet to your ankles, up your calf to your knees. Let the white line stop at every joint. Every part of your body that the white line touches sinks into a deeply relaxed state, feeling heavy and relaxed.

Let the white line move slowly through your legs, into your pelvis, into your back and up your spine; let it split at your shoulders and visualise it running across one shoulder and down one arm to your fingertips and then down the other side.

Pick it up again at the neck and let it move through your neck, over your scalp into your forehead, nose, cheeks, eyes, lips and jaw. Relax your jaw.

Feel your whole body relax deeply. Feel how heavy it is. To move an arm would require a huge effort. Let the words 'deeply, deeply relaxed' go through your mind. Enjoy being relaxed.

When you are ready, slowly, slowly start to come back and slowly open your eyes. Stay there for a few moments and notice how relaxed you feel.

Mindful relaxation

Traditionally, relaxation and meditation have required you to find time and space to practise a combination of breathing, relaxing techniques and emptying your mind of thought. This takes practice and discipline and, above all, it takes time, which busy new parents rarely have.

If you are short on time, or perhaps motivation, this exercise can help to create a relaxing interlude that does not take extra time.

It involves using your everyday activities as rest and relaxation opportunities. You could use washing up, ironing, vacuuming, bathing, gardening or walking as mindfulness exercises. Blow drying your hair or hanging out washing can be useful multi-tasking opportunities. *For safety, it is important that you do not do this exercise while operating potentially dangerous machinery or driving, etc.*

This is the exercise – using washing up as an example (if you can find a way to make washing up relaxing, then why not?) Draw on as many of your senses as possible.

Touch
You can feel your feet on the ground, the drainer against your tummy, your hands in the water.

Sight
You can see the dishes, the water, the kitchen, and perhaps what's going on outside the kitchen window: the grass, the sky, a bird . . .

Hearing
You can hear the noise of the water from the taps, the clinking of the plates, perhaps the TV in the other room, a car going past.

Smell
You can smell the washing-up liquid.

You can also bring in Taste if you are eating; for example, if you are doing the exercise while having coffee and a biscuit.

It is important to be in the present moment, so don't have the radio on and don't go over what has happened or plan what you have to do. Just be involved in the washing up. If your mind wanders, create more noise in the washing-up bowl to bring you back to the present. If you can do the exercise several times a day in different circumstances, so much the better, as it will allow you to have a rest from your over-busy mind.

In addition to relaxation exercises, relaxation can be achieved by finding some me-time and using it constructively (see Chapter 8, What About Me?)

3. Exercising

Exercise relieves any built-up stress hormones in the body and promotes a general relaxation of the nervous system. We all know (we're told often enough!) that exercise is good: physically, it's good for our hearts, our lungs and our circulation; mentally, it's good for our minds and our sense of well-being.

If exercise is this good, then why is it so hard? The evidence seems to be that it is one of those things that the more you do, the easier it gets. And, as with everything, often it's getting started that is the hardest part. Don't run out and buy a gym membership, just try incorporating a little activity into your daily routine. Just twenty minutes, three times a week has proven health benefits.

Here is a pick and mix of activities that count as exercise. Pick the one that suits you at the time.

Skipping

Skipping is a fantastic exercise favoured by top athletes and little girls everywhere. Skip in time to music; skip forwards and backwards, fast and slow. Can you do that one where you cross your arms? Rest as often as you like, but try to spend twenty minutes on the activity.

Roller blading

Could you roller skate as a child? You will probably find you can still do it now, though you may be a bit wobbly at first. Many sports shops sell adult roller blades for as little as £20.

Riding a bike

Do you have a bike? Could you borrow one or look for one secondhand (try Netmums in your area – the Nearly New board can be good for bikes). If you have a toddler, you could think about getting a little seat fitted on the back. Go for a peaceful ride in the summer evenings.

Walking

This certainly isn't a cop out. Walking is wonderful. A study of a pram-walking group in Australia showed that the exercise and the fact that they were with other women helped mums with depression. The mums went three times a week and walked for forty minutes, and their levels of depression decreased. Pick up a pedometer (the price has dropped to around a fiver and you can get them in good chemist's). Aim for 10,000 steps a day, which will include your daily routine and maybe a little bit extra (like walking round the block).

Running

Give yourself a challenge rather than running at random. Can you work out how far a mile is? It might be from your house, round the block and back to your house. Start off walking that mile and time yourself. The next day, walk it a bit faster, then faster. Power walk it. Try to beat your previous time. When you are ready, jog a bit of the way, walk, then jog a bit more. You will be encouraged by how quickly your body adapts and improves its ability to perform. The aim is to be able to run the whole way. If you want to, you can continue to try to beat your time, or maybe you could try doing the circuit twice.

Trampolining

If you are lucky enough to have a garden trampoline, get bouncing – star jumps, turning in midair . . . It is wonderful exercise.

Swimming

A long slow swim can be meditative as well as good exercise. The first few lengths seem hard, but after that you will find you get into the flow. The pool is a great place to think through your problems. Wear goggles so that you aren't straining to keep your head out of the water the whole time, as this can make your neck give up long before the rest of your body does. Let the water bear your weight. Give yourself a targeted number of lengths to do and rest when you need to.

Hoola hoop

Back in fashion (it's the latest fitness craze in Los Angeles), the hoola hoop is great exercise and lots of fun. Not only is it great for fitness, but it works on your waist too.

4. Eating well

What you eat can affect your moods and your mental health and well-being. When we are really down and depressed, often we comfort eat but it doesn't prove comforting at all. In fact, we look at the empty pack of chocolate biscuits and our tight jeans and hate ourselves for not being able to stop. Comfort eating is about trying to fill a gap inside ourselves, but that gap is usually an emotional gap that will never be filled with cakes and biscuits. Can you ask yourself what you are really hungry for? What is that gap inside you? What would you need to fill it? Naming and recognising your real need will perhaps help you to stop trying to fill it with the wrong things.

On the other hand, if you are very stressed or anxious, it can cause you to lose your appetite completely, as your muscles tense up and your body remains on high alert. If you are losing weight and have no appetite, try to eat just a little bit of good, sustaining foods: a slice of brown bread, a bowl of porridge, a banana. And get a supply of good multi-vitamins and take one each day. You need the basic nutrients to help your body and mind overcome this difficult time. You need the energy that foods give you.

Tips

- Don't forget to eat breakfast and make it as substantial as you can. If mornings are a mad rush and you always feel that your time is spent seeing to the children or to your partner, try preparing yourself something the night before.
- Eat slowly; don't bolt down your meals.
- Eat regularly; don't leave it so long between meals that you let your blood sugar levels drop.
- Eat the recommended foods (below) and watch the 'Avoid' foods.
- Plan ahead and stock up on mood boosters. Put together a tin of healthy snacks, e.g. dried-fruit bars, nuts, seeds (even visiting a health food shop can sometimes make you feel better).
- Try shopping online. This helps to avoid the temptation of buying the types of foods that bring your mood down.
- If you are depressed, you may find it difficult to find the enthusiasm to cook or eat properly. Stress also depletes your vitamins and minerals, so take a good multi-vitamin every day.

Foods to Avoid:
Tell yourself, 'This is doing me *no good*' . . .

Refined carbohydrates
These include white bread, white pasta, cakes, sweets and chocolates, and any foods that are high in added sugar. They are bad news for those of us who are trying to stabilise our moods. These foods result in a sudden rise in blood sugar, which gives a quick burst of energy but is followed by a sudden dip in both mood and energy.

Highly processed foods
These typically contain artificial additives and hydrogenated fats. Eating excessive amounts of saturated fats and hydrogenated fats can interfere with the conversion process of the essential fatty acids, which are essential for the brain.

Stimulants
For example, chocolate and caffeine, give you a quick high and then a crashing low.

Alcohol
Drinking alcohol in excess of the Recommended Daily Allowance acts as a depressant, which can make a bad mood worse.

Eat More:
Tell yourself, 'This is *good* for me' . . .

Good carbohydrates
Eating good carbs means eating those with a lower Glycaemic Index (GI). The energy provided by low-GI foods will be released slowly, thus stabilising blood sugar levels, helping you to feel good for longer, and preventing the peaks and troughs of rising and falling

energy levels that may play havoc with your mood.

Foods that fall into this category include: wholemeal breads, boiled potatoes, sweet potatoes, pasta (wholegrain), brown rice, oats, wholegrain cereals.

Protein

As well as an additional source of energy, protein-rich foods provide nutrients, such as iron (especially red meat), B vitamins (needed for nerve function), zinc and magnesium, and the essential amino acids, including tryptophan.

Included in this group are: lean cuts of meat, poultry, fish, eggs, dairy products, such as cheese and milk, nuts (especially walnuts and brazil nuts, which are a good source of selenium), beans (e.g. kidney beans), pulses, such as lentils and chickpeas, and meat substitutes, such as tofu or Quorn.

Fats

Essential fatty acids are so called because they cannot be made by the body and so must be provided by the diet. These fats can be divided into two categories: Omega-6 fatty acids, found predominantly in nuts and seeds, e.g. pumpkin and sunflower seeds; and Omega-3 fatty acids, found in oily fish (sardines, mackerel and salmon). Studies on Omega-3 in particular have shown a relationship between levels of depression and low intakes of the Omega-3 fatty acids. You should aim to include oily fish in your diet twice a week.

Vitamins and minerals

Psychological stress that can lead to or worsen already established depression has been linked to deficiencies in iron, selenium, magnesium, vitamins of the B-complex, folic acid and zinc. Sources of these foods include:

- Iron: red meat, dark-green leafy vegetables, eggs and some fruit, e.g. dried apricots
- Selenium: brazil nuts, liver, kidney, tuna and shellfish, especially crab
- Magnesium: dark-green leafy vegetables, nuts and wholegrains
- B vitamins: wholegrains, yeast
- Folic acid: dark-green leafy vegetables and fortified cereals
- Zinc: wholegrains, legumes (peas, lentils, beans), meat and milk and dairy products.

The antioxidants (vitamins A, C and E) should form part of any healthy and balanced diet. Sources of these nutrients include:
- Vitamin A: liver, milk, cheese and oily fish
- Vitamin C: kiwi, oranges, grapefruit, berry fruits
- Vitamin E: primarily vegetable oils, wheat germ oil, sunflower seeds, peanut butter.

Stop dieting!

Dieting puts stress on an individual and it demands a lot of self-control. This, in turn, results in disturbances in our emotions and can change how we think and feel about ourselves. Adopting a healthy-eating regime is the best way to avoid the pitfalls of stringent dieting and to brighten your outlook for the long term.

See your GP or health visitor

If you are feeling very stressed, or feel you may be even a little depressed, please do go and see your GP. Just because you can't see the symptoms, depression and stress are very real illnesses and your GP will take you seriously.

Tell your doctor all the symptoms that are troubling you – even if you are having scary thoughts. Many women fear admitting these thoughts in case they are judged unfit mothers, but your doctor will not judge you. Scary thoughts are a well-recognised symptom of post-natal depression and doctors know that these thoughts are rarely, if ever, acted upon.

It may be an idea to write down your symptoms and feelings before you go, or see the list in this chapter (see pp. 239–40) and underline or tick the ones that affect you. Many mums find the relief of admitting their feelings causes them to break down in tears when they start talking to their doctor. This is good: the doctor needs to know how you are really feeling to know how best to help you.

A few people find their doctor to be unapproachable or unhelpful. If you are one of them, then go to a different doctor. If you are prescribed anti-depressants, but then decide you don't want to take them, go back and discuss this with your GP. Don't put them in the cupboard and walk away. Talk about all the possible alternatives.

Anti-depressants

Your doctor may suggest anti-depressants. Don't dismiss the idea out of hand. Having young children is hard, but it shouldn't feel impossible. It shouldn't be permanently overwhelming. There should also be happy times – little moments of sunshine that keep us going. If you rarely or never see the sunshine, it can often be because there are not enough *neurotransmitters* in your brain. You've probably heard the names of some of these neuro-transmitters before: serotonin, noradrenalin and dopamine. They are responsible for transferring (or transmitting) messages through the brain, and if their levels drop, the normal messages that prompt good feelings can't get through. Anti-depressants stimulate the increase in the levels of these neurotransmitters. This allows the messages to get through again and helps us to have normal thoughts and reactions.

There is absolutely no shame in taking anti-depressants. Would you take Nurofen or paracetamol for a headache? Would you accept a plaster for a broken arm, or medication for a thyroid imbalance, or an inhaler for asthma? Anti-depressants are not scary drugs that alter your personality or sedate you. Drug treatment for depression and anxiety has come a long way since the days of 'Mother's Little Helper' (Valium, the highly addictive tranquilliser, was the most prescribed drug from 1969 to 1982). You might be surprised to know there are nearly nine million people in the UK taking anti-depressants.

Treatment with anti-depressants these days usually starts with an SSRI (selective serotonin re-uptake inhibitor), such as the infamous Prozac. It takes about ten to fourteen days for the drugs to start working, and six to eight weeks for them to take effect fully. If you don't feel the benefit within that time, see your doctor again and he or she may try a different type – different people respond better to different drugs.

Anti-depressants could be the answer for getting you back on track and back to a place where you can enjoy your children and your life again. If, while you are taking the anti-depressants, you also introduce some of the other effective measures – relaxation, me-time, eating well and so on – by the time you are ready to stop taking them, you'll have built up a stronger internal resource.

Can I breastfeed my baby if I'm taking anti-depressants?

All anti-depressants are secreted in breast milk but the amount that gets into your breast milk is low: about 2 per cent. Generally, there should be no reason why you should stop breastfeeding. Your doctor will be able to advise which type and dosage are best for breastfeeding mothers.

Can I take anti-depressants during pregnancy?

Of the modern drugs, fluoxetine (or Prozac) has been most studied. It has not been shown to cause congenital abnormalities or neurobehavioural effects in children whose mums took it in pregnancy. In summary, there is no evidence of it causing any harm to babies.[2]

(2) This information has been taken from *Drug and Therapeutics Bulletin*, May 2000. Your GP's surgery should have a copy somewhere if you want to know more

10 The Stuff You Can't Legislate For

We've looked at the stresses and strains of everyday life and how we can best manage them. We've realised that although we can't always control what happens in our lives, we can control our responses to what happens. We can't control a flat battery, a toddler tantrum, a moody partner or the proverbial spilt milk, but we can choose how we react to it.

However, life also has a way of throwing other things at us: *big* things that catch us completely off guard and knock us off our well-planned route. Someone once said, 'If you want to make God laugh, tell Him your plans' – and that about sums it up. There are things that happen to us that seem to be life's way of saying, 'Just a reminder that you're not in charge, I am.' These things don't just make us a bit unhappy, they make us truly sad – things such as the death of someone you love, a miscarriage, a relationship breakdown . . . There is nothing that will stop these events from being sad . . . and that is the point. In our pursuit of happiness, we must also factor in that there will be times when we will be sad. Difficult times are a part of life.

The challenge is to get to the stage where we can accept these sad and difficult times, accept that they are a part of growing and developing, a part of our journey through life. At the time, we call out (to God, to the universe, to no one), 'WHY?' but the answer seldom comes. Perhaps when we are old and wise we can look back at this time more philosophically and say that, although we can't understand why it happened, we can at least accept the sadness without anger or bitterness and see that what we have been through has shaped us, has made us what we are. Perhaps it has made us strong. Perhaps it is what taught us patience, humility and empathy with others.

Miscarriage

Miscarriage brings a grief that no one except a woman who has experienced a miscarriage can understand. The depth of our grief is based not on how many weeks pregnant we were, but on how much we had bonded with our baby. And, for most of us, we bond deeply even in the early days. The depth of our grief can seem negated by the medical profession and even family members who say it is normal, common. Others feel sad for us, but many don't view it as the tragedy it is to us. We have lost our baby. We have also lost our dreams, our plans, the birth and the life of that baby. We may wonder if we did something wrong. We may feel we've let our partner down. We grieve deeply but wonder if we should be getting over it more quickly; after all, it's 'just' a miscarriage. And then we have to see other pregnant women and smile, while longing deep within our soul for our own lost pregnancy.

So many people said things like: 'Maybe there was something wrong with the baby. It wasn't meant to be. It's nature's way. You'll have another one.' Inside I was screaming silently at them, 'But I wanted THIS baby, I loved THIS baby – perfect or not.'
Siobhan, Harrow, mum to Sean, 10, Aisling, 7 and Aran, 4

A child with special needs

Shock, anger, devastation, disbelief: these are some of the words mums have used to describe what they felt in the early days of learning their baby or child has special needs. Of course, everyone copes in different ways, and everyone has different sorts of strengths. Some mums can call on strong internal resources to get them through, whereas others crumble and can't face getting out of bed. That is not a sign of strength or weakness – it is just you being the way you are. You can't change your reaction any more than you can change how you react to being at the scene of a car crash: you might have expected yourself to be the calm one who copes and dives in to help, but find yourself instead feeling faint, shaky and crying. Whatever your reaction, whatever your emotions and feelings at this time, you need to accept them and allow them some space. They are real feelings and must be validated.

It is also very much OK to mourn the child that you had wished for and spent nine months preparing for. You had dreams and aspirations for that child. Those dreams need to be gently laid to rest. Many mums feel enormous guilt if they find themselves with negative feelings about their child or about the child's condition or about how unfair it seems. Because you love your child, it may feel like a betrayal to be anything other than delighted, proud, defensive. In many ways, you have lost a child. Even though you have gained a different child, whom you love with a perfect love, you must allow yourself to grieve for your lost child. You can feel that grief without betraying your new, unexpected child.

If you have feelings of anger, or despair, it is important to acknowledge these feelings and not suppress them, as they will come out somewhere else as anger or depression or guilt aimed at the wrong person or thing. Most of all, seek out other parents who have children with similar needs. Talk to them, let them share their stories. They are on the same path as you, though maybe a little further along the road.

> **I have the beauty of having a child who in many ways is enlightened. Joshua is everything we all wish and strive to be, but he has it naturally: he loves life, has no cares, no financial or exam worries. Sometimes I am jealous of his being (if that doesn't seem too weird!) and I realise why I have him. He has a very grounding effect on me and others around him. The future is, of course, a worry, but it seems much brighter than it did at the outset . . . the doom and gloom were so horrific but were soon replaced with such pride. Every milestone is a celebration and even naughty behaviour is 'cute' because he has reached a new stage of learning!**
> **Ruth, Dublin, mum to Joshua, 4, who has Down's Syndrome**

Abortion

For many of us who have found ourselves with an unplanned pregnancy at the wrong time in our lives, abortion is presented as an acceptable option, relatively easy in comparison with having an unwanted child. Abortion is something our doctor, our friends and society in general offer us quite openly, willingly and without judgement.

Even with pre-abortion counselling, some of us are too young, too scared, too confused or too unsupported to see any alternative. Whatever the circumstance of our abortion, there are a great many women who suffer from a deep, silent trauma afterwards.

> **Research from a team in Oslo, published in the** *British Medical Journal* **showed that women who had had an abortion suffered mental distress up to five years and longer after the event. The emotional consequences of having an abortion can be huge, and include anxiety, guilt, flashbacks and depression.**

Mother Teresa once said that the mother who has an abortion is a victim. She believed that a woman who has a baby taken from her womb with her permission would suffer deeply, even if it were deep in her subconscious. She believed that society was to blame for presenting abortion as such an 'easy' option. The point is, she didn't judge the mothers. She pitied them, and she understood the suffering many of them go through.

If you have had an abortion (even though you still feel that abortion was the right thing for you at the time) and you are feeling sadness, guilt or anxiety as a result, it is OK to acknowledge these emotions. Don't suppress them or believe that because it was your choice you have no right to feel this way. Your feelings are real, valid and more common than you think. Many, many women have been and are going through this, and there is help available from people who understand. Start with Care Confidential by calling their freephone number: 0800 028 2228 or www.careconfidential.com.

The loss of a parent

When we become mums, the majority of us still have our mums and dads around too. Even though we may not live nearby, they are still there, still in our lives. Our parents are our final frontier between us and adulthood. Only with our parents can we still be children, their children. And yet as our parents get older, they become less able, less strong. Often they become ill. We find ourselves trying to find time to care for our parents when our hands are already full caring for our children. For this very reason, our generation is known as the 'Sandwich Generation'. In many ways, we start to mourn the loss of our parents even before their death. As they start to weaken, so does our belief in the fact that they will always be there. And this brings the concept of mortality home to us. We know that death exists and we've always known that one day our parents will die. Yet no amount of knowing can prepare you for how it feels to be parted from your mum or dad by death.

We will always miss them. The gap they leave in our life can never be filled . . . we will never 'get over' their death. What we can do is work towards finding a place in our heart for our parents where we can put our love and our memories, and we can carry that place with us through life without pain. But pain is a part of grief and there is no way to avoid it. You need to allow yourself to feel the pain of loss, as the pain is part of the healing.

Spend time remembering your mum or your dad, talking about them, make a photo album and scrapbooks. Don't feel you need to get over it and move on. There is no timescale on grief. Talk to other mums who have lost their parents. Compare your feelings. You will find that what you are going through is very normal and that, in itself, is a comfort.

Of course, not everyone has a great relationship with their parents. If your mother or father was highly critical or demanding, or perhaps worse, unloving and unfeeling towards you, and you have spent your life trying to get their approval and their love, then mixed in with the emotions of grief may be a sense of relief. That feeling of relief lies unacknowledged – it seems like a forbidden feeling and just the idea of it creates guilt, which in turn leads to the suppression of both emotions. Be assured: your feelings are normal and they are acceptable. Allow yourself to feel that relief and to understand why you are feeling it. What would you say to your sister (real or imaginary) if she explained these feelings to you?

The breakdown of a relationship

It certainly wasn't how we'd planned it. We didn't set out to be single mums. We feel we've failed and with that comes the guilt, especially where the children are concerned. It's very human to want to know where to place the blame. It could be your fault or his fault or both, or no one's fault. There are also feelings of bereavement. Even if it was you who instigated the break-up, you are losing someone who was an important part of your life. You have lost your partner, the father of your child, your one-time best friend. Even if you are experiencing relief that a difficult relationship is finally over, you can, at the same time, feel sad and lonely, and you may be afraid of the future. All of these emotions are normal reactions to the breakdown of any relationship. And yet with children involved, the difficulties in a relationship breakdown increase a hundredfold. This is your child's father. He probably wants to remain a big part of your child's life, which means he will stay in your life too. You can't just put him out of your mind and move on.

You want to create an atmosphere of security and normality for your children, but you are falling apart inside. It is good for your children to know at least a little of what you are feeling: wouldn't it perhaps be worse for them to see you unaffected and uncaring? It is normal to be upset and it helps them to validate their own feelings. You need to show them, in part and for a time, that you are sad.

Then there are the other emotions: hate, resentment, anger and jealousy. These are known as the destructive emotions. Talk about these – perhaps to a professional counsellor. This will allow you to acknowledge your feelings and face them without letting them overtake you. Do whatever you need to do to avoid letting these negative emotions bury themselves deep inside you. They are destructive and the people they will hurt are you and your children.

Some ways to help yourself through the difficult times

1. Accept your emotions

We are often afraid of 'big' emotions. They can make us feel out of control and that can be frightening. So we suppress our feelings, but by trying to ignore them, we are pushing them deeper down inside. We may even push them down so deeply that we almost forget they are there. But they will find a way out. They might come out as anger: when we suddenly shout at the children for no good reason. Or depression: when everything should be fine but we feel empty and sad. Or they might come out as anxiety: feeling edgy and nervous even though there is no apparent threat. Or tiredness: the effort of not thinking about something saps energy.

Ask yourself:

Can you name your feelings?

You may find this exercise upsetting, as you are going to take on your negative or anxious feelings. So find a good time and place to do this – not half-an-hour before your favourite TV programme or on a Saturday when you've a shopping trip planned. If you have someone whom you trust and feel you could do the exercise with, then ask her or him to help.

Write down what it is that is causing your anxious feeling; be as detailed and specific as possible. Then name your feeling: anxiety, fear, dread, panic, loss. How big is the feeling? Rate it on a scale of 1 (not much) to 10 (at its worst). Jot down all the thoughts that come into your mind as you become aware of this feeling.

Ask yourself these questions: 'What am I afraid might happen if I allow myself to look more closely at this feeling and the event that causes/caused it? What is the worst thing that can happen if I do choose to look at it more deeply?'

Now, spend some time thinking about the event that causes/caused this feeling. When did it happen? What were the circumstances? Can you go through it in chronological order from beginning to end in your mind? Look at details. What were you wearing? What was the weather like? Who else was there?

Again, once you have written everything down, read over both of your lists and ask yourself: 'Is there a more helpful way that I could think about this event?' Write it down, and then reconsider your initial feeling and how you rated it (1–10). See if you have been able to bring your rating down.

If you have, then well done. If you haven't, then you might have to go over it again to see if you missed something that would have been helpful to you. It might be best if you gave yourself time to think about it before doing the exercise again.

2. Accept good and bad days

The difference between depression and sadness is that in depression you feel no joy, whereas with sadness you can feel even occasional moments of joy. It might be that you are mourning the death of your mother but at the same time laughing with joy at your toddler's new word or your baby's first tooth. This is OK! It is OK to experience very different feelings in the same day. Don't feel guilty because you forgot your sadness for a moment. In fact, rather than waking up and feeling better one day, the usual course will be that you will have an occasional good day with mostly bad days, then a few more good days and a few more, until the bad days get fewer and farther between. Just take it slowly and remember that a bad day does not negate the good days. It doesn't mean you are going backwards. It's just a bad day.

Ask yourself:

How frequent are my bad days?

Keep a daily diary: write a one-line entry each day about how the day was for you. Was it a good day or a bad day? Give it a rating of 1 or 2 for the really black days, 4 for survival, 5 for just OK, 7 for a fairly good day and 9 or 10 for a great day.

This is helpful to look back over on a really black day. On a really bad day, you can't quite believe you will ever feel normal again. But if you look at your diary entries and you can find quite a few good days (look, you even had an 8 last week!) and it is there in your own handwriting, in black and

white, it helps you to believe that you will get through today.
It's simply a bad day.

3. Accept there may not be an answer

Why me? The question can go over and over and round and round
our minds: Why me? Of course you want to look for answers. And
it can help a little to understand the causes behind a miscarriage or
the medical facts behind your father's early death, but after that the
question becomes less helpful. At some stage you may need to
accept that there isn't an answer to this question. Bad things
happen to good people. Stuff happens. Life happens. You haven't
been singled out for something bad. You aren't being punished. It
is a random act of life. It just happened to happen to you.

4. Find something bigger than yourself

When we are desperate for answers, it can be a great comfort to put
our trust in the hands of something or someone bigger than
ourselves. If you have a faith, or had a belief when you were younger
but it lapsed as you got older, now can be a good time to re-examine
and perhaps reawaken your faith. The idea that there is a loving
God (or Buddha or Allah) who knows what it all means and who
cares for us can be a very powerful medicine. Visit a local church or
temple, synagogue or mosque; spend a little time sitting there in
peace and silence. Perhaps ask to speak to the priest, vicar or rabbi?
Read some spiritual books or pamphlets.

5. Find something that takes you out of yourself

Think about the expression 'takes you out of yourself' for a
moment. These are the times we are so busily engaged in
something that we forget about ourselves for a time. We are lost
in our activity. These times give us a break from our over-busy
minds and from our sadness and troubles. This is why people are

known to throw themselves into their work during difficult times. But when looking after little children, although we are fully occupied physically, we are often only half engaged by their constant chit-chat, requests and games, and this give us too much time to think. What takes you out of yourself? Find something each day, even if it is a crossword, Suduko or 1,000-piece jigsaw puzzle. Or borrow a PlayStation or Xbox and blow up some baddies!

6. Take a day at a time

When you are going through difficult times, try not to think too far ahead. Don't think: 'How will I cope with the holidays or Christmas?' Deal with today and what today brings, be it a good day or a bad day. The future can seem overwhelming, but by the time you get to the future it will be the present and you will deal with it as it comes along. Also, you will get stronger every day and you will be at a different stage on your journey when you get to 'the future'. Just deal with today.

7. Get help and support

Your feelings are, of course, unique to you, but there aren't many problems that you will face that haven't been faced by others before you: illness, depression, family problems, relationship issues, addictions. In fact, this is what support groups are: they are formed by, run by and made up of other people who have suffered exactly as you are suffering now. They are all people who didn't expect this problem to happen to them or who didn't expect to react like this. They didn't expect to be helping in this support group either, but they know how lonely and confusing it can be and they want to share their experience with you. There is that expression that says, 'You can't feel my pain until you've walked in my shoes.' These are people who have walked in your shoes.

Your doctor, health visitor or Netmums.com can refer you to your local support group.

8. Acknowledge? Release your inner child

You may have heard of your 'inner child' and dismissed it as pop psychology or psycho-babble, but if you take a moment to think about it you will agree that within each of us is our 'inner child'. This is the childlike part of us, the part that sometimes wants to be silly and giggly, that sometimes doesn't want to be the responsible mum but wants someone else to be in charge, that gets to the seaside and wants to paddle and have an ice cream, or that gets excited about winning at snap and gets competitive at snakes and ladders. Your inner child is the one who still wants to please her parents, who feels anxious before walking into a new group, who feels nervous at the school gate, who maybe sometimes feels scared of the dark. Our inner child is the one who, especially in difficult times, feels that what she really wants is her mum. As an adult, even if your mum is still around, you need more than your mum to care for your inner child. You need your adult self to be able to care for, comfort and mother your inner child.

Where do you start?

Find a quiet time and close your eyes and use the simple relaxation exercise described on pp. 259–60 to help you relax. Now think back to when you were a child, as young as you can remember – somewhere between three and seven years old. Think about how the child looks, how she is dressed, how she does her hair. Think about your childhood home, your bedroom, where you ate your meals. Think about your earliest memories of school: the way it felt, the way it smelt, where you hung your coat. Think about how this child is feeling: is she sad, lonely, scared, worried?

Can you now, in your mind, go to meet that child as your adult self? What is it that your inner child needs to hear? What comfort does she need? Tell her what she needs to hear. Treat her as you would one of your own children if they were upset. And then remember that that child can also be happy, and needs to have some fun and some laughter too. Can you provide that for her? Maybe not today, but can you promise her that there will be fun times ahead? Time spent with your inner child can have long-standing positive effects. Try bringing her out, especially at those times when you feel like shouting, 'I want my mum!'

Final thoughts

Count your blessings

The science of happiness has been studied and measured all over the world by psychologists, psychiatrists, sociologists and all sorts of other clever 'ists'. A key element of being happy that recurs time and time again is the ability to count our blessings, which helps us to focus on the positive instead of the negative. And so, on our continuing quest to be happy mums, try keeping a Happiness Diary. Get yourself a little notebook or pad and entitle it 'My Happiness Diary'. You can write in it at any time of the day but in the evening just before bed might be best, as the feelings you are left with will drift through you while you are asleep.

Day One

On the first page, under day one, write ten things you like about yourself. Don't feel self-conscious: this is your chance to think about the best bits about being you. If you had to write an advert about yourself, what might you say? Are you kind, clever, a good mum, a loyal friend, good fun, thoughtful? If you find it very hard, think about what those closest to you (mum, sister, best friend, partner) might say about you?

Day Two

Write down ten good things you have in your life: people, things, health, work, favourite place, food, sport . . . any ten things that you are grateful to have, things that you would miss if you didn't have them. Think for a minute about what it is you love about each one and why it is important to you.

Day Three

It's food day today. Every time you eat and drink something today, really notice it and think about it. Where did it come from? Wonder about who was involved in its preparation. What was involved in planting it, growing it, tending it, picking it, making it, packing it? Smell and taste your food and drink. Really appreciate it. If you are cooking, think about the ingredients and where they came from. Smell them. Notice how they feel. Enjoy preparing and eating good food. In your Happiness Diary, write a list of the good food you enjoyed today. It's not time to feel guilty if you're on a diet, or didn't eat well enough; think instead of the things you enjoyed eating.

Day Four

In your Happiness Diary today, write down ten things that you have to be thankful for about your health. We rarely notice our good health until we are ill. Remember back to the last time you were sick – perhaps a bug or flu, or perhaps something more serious. You felt awful, were confined to bed, couldn't do any housework or play with the children. Now think about your health: your strong arms, legs, hand, heart. You can talk and laugh. You have a wonderful brain, which is better than hundreds of the most powerful computers. You have your senses: sight, smell, touch, taste, hearing. Appreciate what you have!

Day Five

Today write down the names of ten people you are thankful to have in your life and why. Choose someone from that list that you have been too busy for lately and make a date with them, ideally this week or next. Either invite them round for coffee and cake, arrange to meet for a drink or supper, or settle down when you are fairly sure of a half hour's peace and call them. Perhaps you can 'book' a call with them for the evening and you can both have a glass of wine or hot chocolate while you chat.

Day Six

Today write down ten reasons to be grateful for our abundance of water. Running water is a real privilege and something we often take for granted. Water is life! Think of all the things we use water for without giving it a second thought.

Day Seven

Today read back over the last six days . . . maybe make a few notes, add in something or someone you forgot. Reflect a little on what a lot of things you have to be grateful for: six days, ten things each day – that's sixty things in your life to be grateful for!

Day Eight

In your Happiness Diary, write down ten things that are great about living in this country. We have the NHS: yes, everyone moans about it, but in many countries, like America, it's no money – no treatment, or in the Developing World, no treatment at all. We have education: again, it is much criticised, but we have free education – the guaranteed chance to learn to read and write and learn as much as we want to or are able to. We have freedom to choose our God, and freedom as women. What about things like our countryside? What else do we have to be grateful for about living here? What are *you* most grateful for?

Day Nine

Write down ten wonderful things about each of your children. What are their special personality traits? What are their most lovable moments? Which of their funny little ways really tugs your heartstrings? If you have more than one child, do each one in turn, really focusing on each one in your heart and mind. If you prefer, turn it into a letter to each child starting: 'Dear [child], I love you so much because . . .'

Day Ten

Write down ten things you have to look forward to. It could be something tomorrow, next week, next year or in ten years. It could be simple small things (tonight's supper, the next sunny day, a glass of wine, the next episode of *Doctor Who*) or bigger things (your summer holidays, Christmas, a special family occasion) or long-term dreams (starting your own business one day when the children are older, going away on a long weekend with no children, your daughter's wedding). Really give it some thought.

Day Eleven

Write down ten good things about the weather. Try to challenge that great British pastime of moaning about the weather! But where would we be if we had long-term drought like Africa or a monsoon season? And when did we last appreciate the changing of the seasons – the beauty of autumn, or the excitement of spring, the annual hope of snow at Christmas, the thrill of a thunderstorm or the first really warm day of summer? What is your favourite weather? And can you say something nice about rain?

Day Twelve

In your Happiness Diary, can you write down ten great times you have had together as a family? What about big events: when you found out you were pregnant, your first scan, family holidays or family outings, Christmas? Also include everyday happy moments: the whole family snuggling up on the sofa with duvets on Saturday evenings, your child's first nativity, a family hug? Try to make at least half of them recent events. They don't have to be great occasions; it can often be the smallest things that fix in your heart.

Day Thirteen

Focus on relative wealth. Wealth to a mum in the Developing World is a roof over her head, access to clean water and a goat and two chickens as a food supply. If that mum were to come to your house, she would consider you wealthy beyond her wildest dreams. Can you write down ten things in your house or life that she would consider eye-popping luxury?

Day Fourteen

Play the name-game today. Whether you work full time or are spending today at a toddler group, or even at the supermarket, try to find one person you have never spoken to before. Your aim is to find out their name. Record it in your Happiness Diary: 'I met a new friend called Tina today.'

For me it has been good to make a point of thinking about what is going right, rather than what is going wrong – and being thankful for everything we have. It's so easy to complain about things, e.g. the weather, housework not being done, no free time, etc., but doing this has made me look at life a little differently. Instead of wasting time moaning about things, it makes you think about how you can change things for yourself, and keep that smile on your face for longer!
Rebecca

The thing I noticed the most about doing these tasks was that they forced me to sit down and really think about small things in my life – things that are so easy to take for granted in this materialistic, capitalistic world. I think that is the key to happiness that seems so easy to overlook: pay attention to the stuff that can be easily overlooked and the big stuff will look after itself! Thank you for giving me a reason to remember all the great things in my life.
Shannon

I have found the diary to be a good task that I can keep up with (almost) on a daily basis. It makes me think, brings back good and bad memories and generally allows me a little me-time in a sort of daydream fashion.
Lucian

Epilogue: Pass It On

So, you've read *How to Be a Happy Mum*. Maybe your children aren't perfectly behaved, your house is still untidy and you haven't found five minutes to yourself all week, but at least you have thought about the things you can do to change how you react to life's stresses and strains. And at least you know that you aren't alone. You can dip back into this book at any time for tips, ideas and strategies for coping with what life throws at you.

The final message is to ask you to pass on a little of your new-found happiness. We are always saddened at Netmums by the number of lonely and isolated mums we talk to: mums who gather the courage to go to a toddler group hoping to make a new friend and who come home in silent tears because no one spoke to them; mums who stand at the school gate feeling the loneliest people in the world as everyone else chats in their groups while they stand alone against the back wall; mums who are struggling to keep a brave face when inside they are crumbling with self-doubt and sadness.

None of us ignores these mums on purpose. We are so preoccupied with our buggies, bags and coats, so busy with life that we don't see what is happening to our fellow mums. So, please, let's open our eyes and connect with the mums we pass in our daily lives.

♦ Can you initiate a conversation with another mum whom you have seen around but never or rarely spoken to, whether at the school gates, playgroup, toddler group or at work, in the supermarket, park or shops? Perhaps say how pretty or handsome her child is, ask if the baby sleeps well or where her children go to school, or compliment her shoes, coat, necklace. Just be interested in her. Before you go, ask her name.

♦ Look out for someone who looks possibly lonely or having a bad moment with a screaming child. We all know how awful those moments are. Shoot her a sympathetic smile, or ask if you can help carry her bags. Tell her, 'We've all been there.'

♦ If you go regularly to a toddler group, pre-school, nursery or school, get there five minutes earlier and stand somewhere where you don't normally stand. Look at the group as a whole and watch the arrival of other mums. Start talking to someone who stands apart from the group.

♦ Smile at a stranger. It takes a bit of practice – the first few times you might find yourself smiling a stiff sort of smile – but go for it! Give a nice sunny smile. Don't worry if he or she doesn't smile back; it's sadly so rare these days to be smiled at by a passing stranger that it might take a bit of time to sink in! You never know how far your smile will go . . . it could be just the right moment for the right person.

♦ Find someone who looks left out or uncomfortable. It could be at work that someone is sitting alone at lunchtime while you are all busy gossiping, or there's someone new at toddlers or at your exercise class, or waiting for the children to come out of pre-school or school.

In the Netmums' Coffeehouse forums we regularly hear from mums who feel terribly lonely and who tell us that they try to make new friends but that everyone seems too busy. Perhaps we can be a little less busy and a little more aware of our fellow mums.

Appendix I: Some Direct Selling Companies and Franchisers

Here are just some companies Netmums are familiar with that are offering a franchise or direct selling opportunity suitable for mums who want to work at home. At the time of going to print, these companies are members or pending members of the official associations that govern their industry. However, please do check with the relevant association for up-to-date information.

Further information

1. The British Franchise Association, Thames View, Newtown Rd, Henley-on-Thames, Oxon, RG9 1HG: www.thebfa.org and tel 01491 578050
2. The Direct Selling Association, 29 Floral Street, London, WC2E 9DP: www.dsa.org.uk and tel 020 7497 1234
3. Chat to other mums about their experiences with these and other companies on our 'Working from home' forum at www.netmums.com

Some direct selling companies

Avon Cosmetics Ltd

Avon is probably the most well known of all direct sales companies. You may remember the Avon lady calling in on your own mum! They've modernised a lot in recent years and have some outstanding, very reasonably priced products and a nice catalogue, too.

Address:	Nunn Mills Road, Northampton, NN1 5PA
Tel:	01604 232425
Email:	online contact form
Web:	www.avon.uk.com

Maria says: One of the reasons I decided to become an Avon rep was because I really like the products. But also it means I have to do some exercise at least around three or four times a week. I'm out there, pushing the buggy, dropping off and picking up books and delivering stuff. It helps to keep me on the move and I can make some cash at the same time. Also, you get so addicted to it that you think, 'If I squeeze in one more drop before I have to submit my order, I may get a few more,' which may not give you loads more cash, but does give you a buzz. The only drawback with Avon is when you pick up the books and they are soaked because, yet again, it's been raining.

Lynn says: I am an Avon rep and I am also an Avon sales leader, which means I go out and recruit reps. I have a four-year-old daughter and I fit it around her. Sometimes she comes with me, other times I can do a couple of hours on my own when she is at playgroup. I started when I was pregnant, just doing friends and family and a few homes near where I live. I now have an area of 200 homes and I have recruited 40 reps of my own that I train and support, and I earn commission from them as well. Being a rep means you can pick and choose your own hours and your earnings are unlimited. The more you sell the more you earn.

The Body Shop at Home

'The Body Shop at Home reminds me so much of when I first started out 28 years ago. I wanted a livelihood to help me pay the mortgage. So I did what women are really, really great at – mixing together what they are good at with what interests them to create their own livelihood. Hey presto – The Body Shop was born! Choosing to be a consultant for The Body Shop at Home is much the same. I love the idea that more women can have a career rather than a job, and that women can be free to control their work lives.'
Dame Anita Roddick OBE, founder of The Body Shop and Netmums patron

Address:	Hawthorn Road, Wick, Littlehampton, West Sussex, BN17 7LT
Tel:	08459 05 06 07
Email:	UKOnline.CareCentre@thebodyshop.com
Web:	www.thebodyshop.co.uk

Jayne says: Just wanted to give a quick plug for Body Shop at Home parties. They are great for girlie nights in and stress-free shopping. Choose from pampering, facials and makeovers.I think this is the best job ever. I have only been doing it for two months and wish I'd started sooner

Alison says: Hi, everyone, I am a mother of two and I have been a Body Shop at Home consultant since last November. It is a great job hosting parties and having fun. I get to meet great people and host great parties, with the products I love.

Captain Tortue UK Ltd

A lovely range of clothes for babies and children aged six months to fourteen years that are fashionable, practical, easy to wear, colourful and high quality.

Address:	PO Box 4444, Storrington, West Sussex, RH20 3WY
Tel:	01903 74 44 44
Email:	info.uk@captain-tortue.com
Web:	www.captain-tortue.com

Razia says: Join us at Captain Tortue selling high-quality children's clothes through private sales in the home. Start-up costs are low, the role fits around your family, with free training and support. You need to be self-motivated, well presented, excited by children's fashion and enjoy socialising.

Creative Memories

Teach others how to preserve those memories by organising that stack of photos that we all have lurking in a drawer somewhere, and there's the added bonus of sorting your own out at the same time!

Address:	9 Pipers Lane Estate, Thatcham, Berks, RG19 4NA
Tel:	01635 294700
Email:	info@creativememories.com
Web:	www.creativememories.co.uk

Kimberley says: I started last January and am LOVING it! I am a Scrapbook Consultant. I go to people's houses and teach them how to preserve their memories into safe, acid-free albums. Our mission is to get people's photos out of shoeboxes and get them into the albums. We call these 'strangers in a box'.

Valerie says: The whole idea behind Creative Memories is to preserve memories for future generations through keepsake albums. All products are totally safe to use with your photos. I've been a Creative Memories consultant for over two years, but a customer for nearly four. I am currently working on five albums, recording the special times my family and I share. I find that working on my album at local workshops provides me with me-time, a time to relax and remember the times that have past, through my photos, as well as having a coffee and sharing ideas with other 'memory makers'. Creative Memories has brought something so special and rewarding into my life. As a consultant I offer home classes, twice-monthly workshops (the first one is free), supplies and support to my customers.

Demarle Ltd

Direct selling quality French Kitchen tools through home cookery workshops.

Address:	1st Floor, 21 Dartmouth Street, Westminster, London, SW1H 9BP
Tel:	020 7304 7092
Email:	consultants@demarle.ltd.uk
Web:	www.demarle.com

Claire says: I work part time for Demarle Ltd, a French company, and am my own boss. I have no targets to reach, just very attractive incentives which are there to motivate, but no pressure is given. The workshops are informative, sociable and tons of fun to be part of – we get everyone to participate in creating a couple of recipes, then they all sample the yummy results at the end! It's female bonding in the kitchen with some unique quality products, which have changed my life in the kitchen as they cut out the mess and the washing up and bring out the creative in us all.

ENJO UK

Alternative body care products.

Address:	Unit C7, Elstree Business Centre, Elstree Way, Borehamwood, Herts WD6 1RX
Tel:	0870 900 6600
Email:	office@enjo.co.uk
Web:	www.enjo.co.uk

Tracy says: Being an ENJO consultant has changed my life. I have been a very happy housewife and mother of three fantastic children for twenty years. Believe me, it was very hard to start my own business and a new career. There are so many positives in what I do. I still have time to watch my teenage children at their individual sporting and school events, etc., which is important to me. Working from home lets me live a very full life of my own when the children don't need me. ENJO has given me a great career path, income, self-belief, overseas travel and a new way of life. I know that ENJO is making a difference in the world. I am very proud of being a part of the ENJO UK family.

Nicky says: ENJO has changed my life! Not only have I found the solution to cleaning without chemicals, with fantastic results, but I was so impressed with the ENJO fibre technology system that I joined a growing team of consultants. Now I show other people that there is an alternative way of cleaning, using water, which is quick, easy, economical and lasts ages. Hard to believe, easy to use! ENJO wants to change the perception of cleaning, so we do demonstrations in people's homes, which are fun as well as informative. For me, ENJO ticks all the boxes – fits in around my family commitments, I get great training and team support, and I know that what I am doing is worthwhile in terms of the health of my family, my career prospects and being environmentally responsible. Together we can make a difference!

Kleeneze

Very useful home-cleaning products.

Address:	St Ivel Way, Tower Road North, Warmley, Bristol, BS30 8TY
Tel:	08703 33 66 88
Email:	service.centre@kleeneze.co.uk
Web:	www.kleeneze.co.uk

Vanessa says: I work from home running a Kleeneze business, and have been doing so for a couple of months now. It is really easy. You just deliver the catalogues to friends/family/groups and collect them in with the orders that people want to place. Once they are delivered to you, you simply take the orders to the customers. I have found Kleeneze to be a very professional company to work with and they provide constant support and guidance to help you get started. I have only done about eight–ten hours a week for the last eight weeks but have already made a fair sum, which has helped me out no end. It is also something I can do mostly when my little boy has gone to bed, so the time I do get to spend with him isn't interrupted.

Mary Kay Cosmetics (UK) Ltd

A wide range of cosmetic and body-care products. Mary Kay is the number-one cosmetic company in America and is growing fast over here.

Address:	28 Savile Row, London, W1S 2EU
Tel:	0800 318 288
Email:	Cserviceuk@mkcorp.com
Web:	www.marykay.co.uk

Miglio

Miglio sells unique designer South African jewellery that incorporates beautiful Swarovski crystals.

Address:	Henhayes House, 29a Market Street, Crewkerne, Somerset, TA18 7JU
Tel:	01460 279960 and 0845 430 9045
Email:	info@miglio.co.uk
Web:	www.miglio.co.uk

Inyang says: Fantatstic company to work for and very fulfilling to be a Miglio consultant.

Mini IQ

Mini IQ brings to you a range of fun, interactive and educational books, toys and games to help support children's development.

Address:	Greater London House, Hampstead Road, London, NW1 7TZ
Tel:	0845 650 2044
Email:	enquiries@mini-iq.co.uk
Web:	www.mini-iq.co.uk

Sue says: I am a mum to two children under three. I sell Mini IQ books, toys and games as a Party Plan and love it. Not only do I get to spend all day with my children, I also get to buy my items at ridiculously low prices and earn some money into the bargain. I really enjoy the meeting people side of Mini IQ. It has become my social life and I love people's reactions to the great products. Everyone loves the quality and individuality of the products – all of which are educational as well as fun and interactive. They really do sell themselves. I have just started to build up a team, but you can really do as little or as much as you like. It is part of my life now (my way of clinging to sanity!) and I've not regretted my decision to become a Mini IQ associate for one minute!

Oriflame UK Ltd

A Swedish beauty and cosmetics company selling its products in over 55 countries through a network of direct sales representatives. Its original business concept is 'Natural Swedish Cosmetics from Friend to Friend'.

Address:	PO Box 57, Leeds, West Yorkshire, LS14 1XG
Tel:	0845 44 44 02
Email:	info@oriflame.org.uk
Web:	www.oriflame.org.uk

The Pampered Chef UK Ltd

Slightly more upmarket kitchen products to bring out the domestic goddess in you! You can apply to be a direct selling agent and then perhaps host a kitchen show or cooking demonstration!

Address:	3 Cheapside Court, Buckhurst Road, Ascot, Berkshire, SL5 7RF
Tel:	01344 293 900
Email:	vi.moore@pamperedchef.com
Web:	www.pamperedchef.com

Nina says: I went to a Pampered Chef demo five years ago and then became a consultant because it looked like fun, and the idea of being my own boss really appealed. I'd given up my career to stay at home with my babies and the idea of doing the part-time jobs I'd done as a student years before or having to work weekends was not what I wanted. I felt it was impossible to find a part-time job I could be proud of and then, thank goodness, Pampered Chef appeared. I was pleasantly surprised by all the training and support offered to me, as well as incentive luxury trips and the career potential of the business. Five years on and my business has grown. Both my children are now at school full time and I'm under no pressure to go back to my old social services career. What this really means is that not only am I now earning significantly more than in my previous, very stressful job, but I have no problems with half-terms, nativity plays, assemblies, sports days. For me, the biggest benefit is being able to help out in my children's classes and have peace of mind as to how they are doing/enjoying school.

Partylite UK Ltd

Direct sales marketer of a very posh range of candles and accessories that you can sell by having candle parties or a stand at school fairs and fêtes.

Address:	Argyle House, Joel Street, Northwood Hills, Pinner, Middx, HA6 1NS
Tel:	01923 848730
Email:	info@uk.partylite.com
Web:	www.partylite.co.uk

Jane says: I just thought I'd take this opportunity to tell you all about Partylite candles. As a consultant it's fantastic. It costs nothing to join, the kit is free, there is no pressure to sell, and it's great fun. The main reason I signed up was to get the £300 worth of kit free, but I love it so much I am staying on.

Phoenix Trading

A huge range of quality greeting cards, wrapping paper, stationery and accessories that practically sell themselves. After all, everyone always needs cards for all those parties that the children get invited to!

Address:	Unit 6, 307–309 Merton Road, London, SW18 5JS
Tel:	020 8875 9944
Email:	info@phoenix-trading.co.uk
Web:	www.phoenix-trading.co.uk

Ragged Bears Publishing

A variety of fun and educational books, toys and games for children, supporting the National Curriculum. Ragged Bears offers an opportunity for parents to run a business around their family.

Address:	Unit 14a, Bennetts Field Trading Estate, Southgate Road, Wincanton, Somerset, BA9 9DT
Tel:	01963 34300
Email:	rblj.wincanton@virgin.net
Web:	www.raggedbears.co.uk

Usborne Books at Home

Usborne, one of the UK's top children's publishers, also uniquely offers a business opportunity throughout the UK and Europe selling through school-book fairs, home parties and other bookselling events.

Address:	Unit 8, Oasis Park, Eynsham, Witney, Oxon, OX29 4TU
Tel:	01865 883731
Email:	mail@usbornebooksathome.co.uk
Web:	www.usbornebooksathome.co.uk

Angela says: I have just become an Usborne Books organiser, selling books for children aged from birth to sixteen years. I am really enjoying it and the books are selling well. I have two three year olds and didn't want to go back to work. This way I can go to mother and toddler groups, show my books and the children come with me! You get a lovely starter kit full of books and stationery for a very low cost.

Nicola says: I've been an Usborne Books organiser for three years now. I began before my son started school and used it as a way of buying books for him at a discounted price and earning a bit of extra cash. Since he's started school it has become so much more and I now have a small team of people who also sell the books. For me it's the best job in the world. I work when I want to, meet lots of people and have *loads* of great books. I've also made lots of new friends, go to fab company events and have lots of fun.

Jenny says: I have just become an organiser for Usborne Books. It's great fun and I love it. The start-up cost is low and there are no targets to meet.

Susan says: I have just started being an Usborne Books organiser and didn't realise what lovely books they are! They don't just sell baby and toddler books, but books for teenagers, too, as well as jigsaws and much, much more! What are you waiting for?

Virgin Vie at Home

Award-winning products, great earning potential, exciting incentives and all backed by Sir Richard Branson. This is a cosmetics and jewellery company with the refreshing Virgin approach.

Address:	Salisbury House, City Fields Business Park, Tangmere, Chichester, West Sussex, PO20 6FP
Tel:	0845 300 80 22
Email:	services@virgincosmetics.com
Web:	www.virginvieathome.com

Rachel says: I started as a Christmas consultant for Virgin Vie last year but was soon hooked. To join only for Christmas is a great way to start because it is cheaper and you only need to do it for a little while – a sort of toe-in-the-water test. It is the perfect job for me as it tops up my wages from my boring day job and gives me flexibility around my beautiful two year old.

Lucy says: I am happily building my Virgin Vie business and really can't sing enough praises about my job. It is fantastic working around my gorgeous daughter's schedule! I'm hoping to try for another baby early next year and so want to ditch my boring job and work for myself with Virgin Cosmetics and Virgin Jewellery so that I can spend more time at home. I would recommend it to anybody else.

Some Franchisers

Gymboree Play and Music UK

The joy of helping children develop and grow . . . is this the career for you? More than just a mother/toddler group or play gym, the Gymboree programme consists of a range of eight curriculum-based classes (plus birthday parties!) that you can present within your dedicated geographical area. This highly flexible franchise enables you to tune the business to your personal demands and the local market. Over 400 worldwide franchisees, thirty years' experience and a dedicated and skilled UK support system.

Address:	8 Shepherd Market, Unit 127, London, W1J 7JY
Tel:	Martin Lawson, direct line: 0777 3333 144 Head Office: 020 7258 1415
Email:	info@gymboreeplayuk.com
Web:	www.gymboree-uk.com

Jo Jingles Ltd

Music, singing and movement classes for children aged six months to five years with a series of varied educational programmes.

Address: 1 Bois Moor Road, Chesham, Bucks, HP5 1SH

Tel: 01494 778989

Email: headoffice@jojingles.co.uk

Web: www.jojingles.co.uk

Kumon Maths and English

Individualised after-school study programmes designed to help children of all ages and abilities to fulfil their potential in maths and English.

Address: Regional Offices in Bristol, Glasgow, London, Manchester and Nottingham.

Tel: 0800 854 714

Email: online enquiry form

Web: www.kumon.co.uk

Little Impressions Ltd

Using a simple and quick clay-moulding technique, create lasting impressions of children for parents, grandparents, godparents or friends to enjoy forever.

Address: Unit 36, Brunel Way, Segensworth, Fareham, Hants, PO15 5SA

Tel:	01489 579 538
Email:	tonyf@little-impressions.com
Web:	www.little-impressions.com

Monkey Music Limited

Introducing music to very young children in a way they can understand and enjoy.

Address:	Unit 3, Thrales End Lane, Thrales End Farm, Herts, AL5 3NS
Tel:	01582 766464
Email:	jointheteam@monkeymusic.co.uk
Web:	www.monkeymusic.co.uk

Nippers

The shop for mums-to-be.

Address:	Little Porters, Porters Lane, Fordham Heath, Colchester, CO3 9TZ
Tel:	01206 241116
Email:	enquiries@nippers.co.uk
Web:	www.nippers.co.uk

SportsCoach

Providing children aged between six and sixteen years with the most exciting, educational and exhausting three hours of their week!

Address:	The Courthouse, Elm Grove, Walton-on-Thames, Surrey, KT12 1LZ
Tel:	01932 256262
Email:	info@scoach.co.uk
Web:	www.sportscoach.co.uk

Stagecoach Theatre Arts plc

Part-time performing arts schools for young people aged between four and sixteen.

Address:	The Courthouse, Elm Grove, Walton-on-Thames, Surrey, KT12 1LZ
Tel:	01932 254333
Email:	mail@stagecoach.co.uk
Web:	www.stagecoach.co.uk

Tumble Tots (UK) Ltd

Structured physical play sessions for pre-school children helping to develop balance, co-ordination and agility skills and developing language through music, action songs and rhymes.

Address:	Bluebird Park, Bromsgrove Road, Hunnington, Halesowen, West Midlands, B62 0TT
Tel:	0121 585 7003
Email:	info@tumbletots.com
Web:	www.tumbletots.com

Appendix II: Some Useful Addresses

Adders.org
A website that provides an insight on ADD/ADHD, as well as providing information, links and more on ADD and related disorders.

Tel: 0870 9503693

Email: support@adders.org

Web: www.adders.org.uk

Barnardos
A leading UK children's charity supporting 100,000 children and their families.

Tel: 020 8550 8822

Email: dorothy.howes@barnardos.org.uk

Web: www.barnardos.org.uk

Child Death Helpline, The
A helpline for those affected by the death of a child.

Tel:	0800 282986
Email:	contact@childdeathhelpline.org
Web:	www.childdeathhelpline.org.uk

Children's Information Service
Provides a service to parents who wish to make enquiries about child-care and education.

| Email: | childcarelink@opp-links.org.uk |
| Web: | www.childcarelink.gov.uk/index.asp |

Citizens Advice Bureau
Practical and up-to-date advice on a wide range of issues including debt, employment, housing and benefits.

| Web: | www.adviceguide.org.uk |

Care Confidential
Help for those facing an unplanned pregnancy, or with post-abortion concerns.

Tel:	0800 028 2228
Email:	admin@careconfidential.com
Web:	www.careconfidential.com

Contact a Family
The leading UK charity supporting families with disabled children.

Tel:	0808 808 3555
Email:	conditions@makingcontact.org
Web:	www.cafamily.org.uk

Criminal Records Bureau
Helps organisations in the public, private and voluntary sectors by identifying candidates who may be unsuitable to work with children or other vulnerable members of society.

| Tel: | 0870 90 90 811 |
| Web: | www.crb.gov.uk |

Cry-sis
Offers support for families with excessively crying, sleepless and demanding babies.

Tel:	08451 228 669
Email:	info@cry-sis.org.uk
Web:	www.cry-sis.org.uk

Disabled Parents Network
A membership organisation of and for disabled parents.

Tel:	08702 410 450
Email:	e-help@disabledparentsnetwork.org.uk
Web:	www.disabledparentsnetwork.org.uk

Down's Syndrome Association
Supports people with Down's Syndrome and their families.

Tel:	0845 230 0372
Email:	info@downs-syndrome.org.uk
Web:	www.dsa-uk.com

Family Links
Promotes nurturing and emotional well-being, building family relationships through workshops.

Tel:	01865 401800
Email:	info@familylinks.org.uk
Web:	www.familylinks.org.uk

Fathers Direct
National centre on Fatherhood.

| Tel: | 0845 634 1328 |

| Email: | mail@fathersdirect.com |
| Web: | www.fathersdirect.com |

FlyLady

Offers tips, advice and humour on keeping your home neat and tidy.

| Web: | www.flylady.net |

Gingerbread

Gingerbread is the leading support organisation for lone parent families in England and Wales.

Tel:	0800 018 4318
Email:	office@gingerbread.org.uk
Web:	www.gingerbread.org.uk

Home-Start UK

Supporting families with children under five years old.

Tel:	0800 068 63 68
Email:	info@home-start.org.uk
Web:	www.home-start.org.uk

I CAN

I CAN is the charity that helps children with speech and language difficulties across the UK.

| Tel: | 0845 225 4071 |
| Web: | www.ican.org.uk |

International Au Pair Association

An international community and trade association specialising in providing culture exchange services. Member organisations must meet certain business and ethical standards.

| Web: | www.iapa.org |

La Leche League GB
Offering support and advice about breastfeeding.

Tel:	0845 456 1855
Email:	admin@laleche.org.uk
Web:	www.laleche.org.uk

National Autistic Society
Providing information and support.

Tel:	0845 070 4004
Email:	nas@nas.org.uk
Web:	www.nas.org.uk

National Childbirth Trust
Offers support in pregnancy, childbirth and early parenthood.

Tel:	0870 444 8707
Email:	enquiries@national-childbirth-trust.co.uk
Web:	www.nct.org.uk

National Childminding Association
Promotes quality home based childcare.

Tel:	0845 880 0044
Email:	info@ncma.org.uk
Web:	www.ncma.org.uk

National Council for One Parent Families
Supports lone parents in England and Wales.

Tel:	0800 018 5026
Email:	info@oneparentfamilies.org.uk
Web:	www.oneparentfamilies.org.uk

National Family Mediation

Offers mediation help to couples, married or unmarried, in the process of separation or divorce.

Tel: 01392 271610

Email: general@nfm.org.uk

Web: www.nfm.org.uk

NHS Direct

Offers medical advice if you're unsure whether to see a GP or not.

Tel: 0845 4647

Web: www.nhsdirect.nhs.uk

One Parent Families Scotland

Works on behalf of lone parents and their families since 1944.

Tel: 0808 801 0323

Email: info@opfs.org.uk

Web: www.opfs.org.uk

Parentline Plus

National Helpline offering Parent to Parent support.

Tel: 0808 800 2222

Web: www.parentlineplus.org.uk

Parent's Partnership

Provides information and support to parents of children with Special Educational Needs.

Tel: 020 7843 6058

Web: www.parentpartnership.org.uk

Recruitment and Employment Confederation
Represents recruitment professionals, businesses and agencies in the UK.

Web: www.rec.uk.com

Relate
The Relationship People.

Tel: 0845 456 1310 or 01788 573 241

Web: www.relate.org.uk

Samaritans
Open twenty-four hours, every day to befriend and support those going through personal crises.

Tel: 08457 90 90 90

Email: jo@samaritans.org

Web: www.samaritans.org

The Baby Café
Drop in centres offering advice and support for breastfeeding mothers and families.

Email: admin@thebabycafe.co.uk

Web: www.thebabycafe.co.uk

Women's Aid
Helping women suffering from domestic violence.

Tel: 0808 2000 247

Email: helpline@womensaid.org.uk

Web: www.womensaid.org.uk

Index

You can buy any of these other titles in the **netmums** series from your bookshop or direct from the publisher.

FREE P&P AND UK DELIVERY
(Overseas and Ireland £3.50 per book)

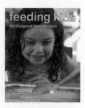

FEEDING KIDS *Netmums with Judith Wills* £14.99

Feeding Kids includes 120 easy-to-prepare and delicious recipes provided by Netmums members that will fit perfectly into your busy family life.

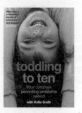

TODDLING TO TEN *Netmums with Hollie Smith* £12.99

Toddling to Ten looks at fifty of the most common parenting problems – from ditching the dummy to beating bullying – and offers expert advice to help you combat them along with the personal stories from the Netmums themselves.

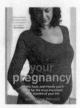

YOUR PREGNANCY *Netmums with Hilary Pereira* £12.99

Your Pregnancy is an invaluable source of mum-to-mum insights and practical know-how from Netmums members, which will make you feel as though you have your very own antenatal group in the comfort of your home.

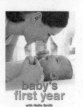

BABY'S FIRST YEAR *Netmums with Hollie Smith* £12.99

Baby's First Year is packed with peer-to-peer guidance and tips from the members of Netmums as well as key medical and developmental information from the experts to help you through the first crucial months of your baby's life.

To order, simply call 01235 400 414
visit our website: www.headline.co.uk
or email orders@bookpoint.co.uk

Prices and availability are subject to change without notice.

To become part of the Netmums community, log on to www.netmums.com.

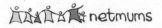